Essential Knowledge and Skills for Healthcare Assistants

Essential Knowledge and Skills for Healthcare Assistants

Zoë Rawles BN RGN BSc (Hons) Nurse Practitioner
Independent Nurse Practitioner
Director/Trainer for HealthTrain www.healthtrain.co.uk

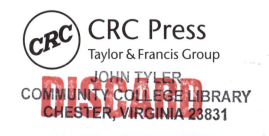

CRC Press
Taylor & Francis Group

CRC Press
Taylor & Francis Group
6000 Broken Sound Parkway NW, Suite 300
Boca Raton, FL 33487-2742

© 2014 by Taylor & Francis Group, LLC
CRC Press is an imprint of Taylor & Francis Group, an Informa business

No claim to original U.S. Government works

Printed on acid-free paper
Version Date: 20131121

International Standard Book Number-13: 978-1-4441-6923-2 (Paperback)

Library of Congress Cataloging-in-Publication Data

Rawles, Zoe, author.
  Essential knowledge and skills for healthcare assistants / Zoe Rawles.
  p. ; cm.
  Includes bibliographical references and index.
  ISBN 978-1-4441-6923-2 (pbk. : alk. paper)
  I. Title.
  [DNLM: 1. Nurses' Aides--standards--Great Britain. 2. Nurse's Role--Great Britain. 3. Primary Health Care--methods--Great Britain. WY 193]

RT84
610.7306'98--dc23   2013045714

Visit the Taylor & Francis Web site at
http://www.taylorandfrancis.com

and the CRC Press Web site at
http://www.crcpress.com

Contents

Foreword

Essential Knowledge and Skills for Healthcare Assistants (HCAs) is a most welcome addition to the small number of textbooks available for HCAs. It covers vital aspects that all HCAs need to know, including accountability, communication and confidentiality to name a few.

The book also explains many practical activities that are relevant to most HCAs, in particular those working in the primary-care setting. Urinalysis, lung function testing and promoting health are included amongst many other key interventions. The practical skills sections are supplemented by essential underpinning knowledge, which will help to broaden the reader's understanding of not only how, but why certain tests and activities are performed.

The importance of patient-centred care is reinforced throughout, as is the necessity for robust protocols covering all roles that HCAs perform. Each section is concise and relevant for HCAs at every stage of their development. This will be a key reference text to support programmes of education and should be on every GP practice's bookshelf.

A nurse practitioner with many years' experience, Zoë Rawles has been involved in the education and training of HCAs since 2003. She has also lectured on the nurse practitioner master's course at the University of Wales Swansea and coauthored a book on physical examination procedures for advanced nurses and independent prescribers in 2010.

Zoë has a talent for explaining complex issues in a clear and uncomplicated way, and draws on her wide experience to illustrate the text with plenty of examples to bring the concepts to life. The book is easily readable yet packed with useful information. Any HCAs who read this book will gain a real understanding of their role and what should be expected of them in practice.

Tanis Hand
HCA Adviser, Royal College of Nursing

Acknowledgements

My thanks to my long-suffering husband John for his support and for putting up with my long absences during the writing of this book. Thanks also to my illustrator, Lucy, for striving to comply with my every whim and request!

Introduction

This book is the result of many years of involvement with the training of health-care assistants (HCAs) and a realisation that most of the books available are aimed more at HCAs working in secondary care. Inevitably this has been aimed more at HCAs working in primary care as this is my area of work and expertise, but it will undoubtedly be a useful resource for HCAs working in other areas as well. There are many different titles for HCAs as discussed in Chapter 1, but for the purposes of this book the term HCA will be used from here on.

The book covers some of the more theoretical aspects of the role but also endeavours to provide an accessible and "user-friendly" approach to learning some of the underpinning knowledge and practical tasks that are now routinely included in the job description of the HCA. It does not assume a level of knowledge but starts at the grassroots and describes the appropriate skills required for levels 2+3 on the Career Framework outlined by *Skills for Health* (2010). These are equivalent to GCSE (grades C-A*) and A-levels, respectively. At this level you, as the HCA, are performing tasks that are delegated to you under supervision from registered professionals. You should act according to clear protocols at all times and must demonstrate competence supported by the required level of knowledge before being delegated particular tasks (RCN 2011). You should not be expected to make a clinical assessment of the patient or make clinical decisions by yourself. Throughout the book there are constant reminders of the need for a protocol for every task and the information provided in each chapter can be utilised and adapted for developing protocols. Wherever possible, the techniques described are based on current national guidelines and are in line with National Occupational Standards (*Skills for Health* 2011) and referenced accordingly. The book does not replace accredited training but does provide an essential resource for those of you who are currently undergoing such training at Levels 2+3.

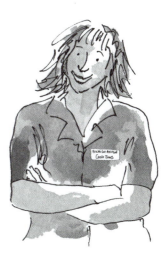

Please read the chapters and engage in the activities and quizzes to reinforce your learning.

I hope you will enjoy developing your understanding about the amazing human body and discover how you can develop your own role and assist in the monitoring and promotion of health for your patients.

Author Biography – Zoë Rawles

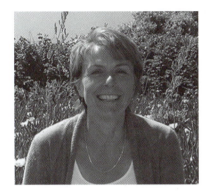

Zoë qualified as a nurse in 1980, having trained in one of the first nursing degree courses in the country, and she graduated from the Welsh National School of Medicine in 1980. She then worked in a hospital on an ENT and orthopaedic ward but soon realized that her real interest lay in the community setting. From then until the present day, Zoë has lived in Wales and worked in the community or in general practice with a few years' break to have three amazing children. In 1999 she graduated as a nurse practitioner from Swansea University with a First Class Honours Degree and subsequently worked as a lecturer on the same course from 2001 to 2009 during its transition from a degree to master's course. In 2009 to 2010 she co-wrote the book *Physical Examination Procedures for Advanced Nurses and Independent Prescribers* with two colleagues.

In 2003 while working in general practice, Zoë mentored healthcare assistants who were undergoing a training course and she became very interested in the developing role. She set up a business (HealthTrain) with a nursing colleague and developed accredited training for primary-care staff including healthcare assistants. Zoë has been running the business singlehandedly since 2009, and it goes from strength to strength offering a range of accredited training packages to HCAs and other primary-care staff all over the country.

Lucy Freegard, Illustrator

Lucy is a freelance illustrator living in London. She graduated with a First Class Honours Degree in illustration and won the Illustration Dissertation of the Year Award from Cardiff School of Art and Design in 2012. She enjoys drawing people and works spontaneously with an expressive and loose approach, giving a sense of movement, expression, and gesture.

Section I
All Change

Evolving Role of the Healthcare Assistant (HCA)

Healthcare assistants (HCAs) have been very much in the background for many years but are increasingly being used at the frontline of healthcare. The development of the role in recent years has been exponential and left some nurses shaking their heads in disbelief and asking if their own role is being eroded at a similar rate. Other nurses have embraced the role with open arms, regarding it as an opportunity to develop their own role and broaden their skills in other more complex areas.

It is difficult to establish exactly where and when the HCA role started to appear on the scene. It may be associated with the demise of the state-enrolled nurse (SEN) role and the subsequent gap in the task force for more "hands-on" capable nurses who are willing to do the more practical tasks. It may also be associated with the rise in degree-led training for nurses, with the commonly held belief, right or otherwise, that nurses trained at such a level no longer want to engage in the more practical tasks so essential to holistic nursing care. Some would even go so far as to say that this degree training does not equip nurses adequately for these tasks. As a nurse who trained on one of the very first degree courses from 1976 to 1980, I am all too familiar with the arguments that rage around this topic and cannot agree with them, having been fortunate enough to see it from the other side.

So what other reasons can there be for the emergence of the role, and where did it all start?

Support workers and HCAs can actually be found as far back as the Crimean War and the role of the auxiliary nurse was then established in 1955 (Kessler et al. 2010). The NHS & Community Care Act (1990) formally recognised the HCA role, introducing it as a role to complement the existing nursing auxiliary role. Support workers have since been adopted to a greater or lesser extent in every area of health and social care. The Royal College of Nursing (RCN) has recognised the importance of support workers as providing a large proportion of hands-on care in many different settings and has described them as "valued and integral members of the nursing team" (RCN 2012a). This is quite a leap forward from when I began my nursing career in 1980. I can remember some extraordinarily capable SENs and nursing auxiliaries in my early nursing days, but I only became aware of the healthcare assistant role in the mid-1990s. The practice I worked for felt that there was a need for a member of staff to be specifically employed to assist in taking blood pressure and other physiological measurements, as well as performing various administrative tasks that were historically part of the practice nurse role. These were considered to be tasks that were an inappropriate use of the practice nurse's skills and time. The General Practitioner (GP) Contract was also emerging at this time and practice nurses started to move away from the treatment room and were given responsibility for more chronic disease management. We then needed someone capable of performing the essential treatment room tasks such as phlebotomy and taking blood pressure. A member of the reception staff was duly sent on the only available course for HCAs that was available at the time, and I was asked to be her mentor. This was the start of my long and happy acquaintance with the HCA role. Together with a practice nurse colleague, I became very interested in the emerging role, and we quickly realised that the training provided was very patchy and in most places was non-existent with little ongoing support for newly trained HCAs. We developed accredited training courses and refresher courses for HCAs and began to understand the full potential of this new and exciting role on the nursing team.

Other factors that have been identified as driving forces behind the rise of the HCA role have been outlined in a review of the evidence by the NHS for Scotland (2010): these include increasing pressure on primary and secondary healthcare systems caused by the ageing population, advances in medical treatments, increasing costs of delivering healthcare, increasing patient expectations, and shortages of qualified healthcare staff. The rise in chronic diseases and continued reduction in the length of hospital stays, with the subsequent effect on primary and community care, have also been cited.

WHY SHOULD HCAs BE REGULATED?

As word spread about reception staff becoming HCAs and performing phlebotomy, blood pressure measurements, and numerous other clinical and administrative tasks, new HCAs began to spring up everywhere in primary (and secondary) care. Kessler et al. (2010) estimated the numbers of those defined as support workers who support clinical staff, as 284,000 in England in 2008. It could only be an estimate because of the continuing confusion over the various titles in use, but nevertheless the group constituted a significant percentage of the NHS workforce then and has been steadily increasing ever since.

Despite this, many HCAs and registered nurses still appeared to be either very unsure or else completely unaware of the issues around appropriate delegation and accountability and the need for accredited training and robust protocols. From my own experience, whilst training HCAs throughout Wales and England, I know that this is still very much the case. The Nursing and Midwifery Council (cited in the RCN Position statement on the education and training of HCAs 2012a) commissioned a study in 2010, which identified that healthcare support workers undertake tasks for which they are not trained; tasks which should be carried out under the direction of a registered practitioner are performed unsupervised; and deployment may depend on staffing levels, trust policies, and perceptions of registered staff, rather than on qualifications and competence of healthcare support workers. There does however, seem to be an increasing awareness of the issues. The NHS in Wales has introduced a code of conduct for support workers and a code of practice for employers (Welsh Assembly Government 2011). Scotland has also introduced similar codes accompanied by mandatory induction standards (Scottish Government 2010). England is lagging behind a little but work is underway on a similar code of conduct with a proposal due to be published. Unfortunately in England there will be no corresponding code for employers setting out their responsibilities. Without the employers' support it will be difficult for support workers to comply with codes of conduct or access induction standards and core competencies.

Titles are a difficult and an ongoing cause of confusion within the profession and amongst the general public. There are many different titles essentially describing the same role, including healthcare assistant, healthcare support worker, clinical-support worker, care-team assistant, nursing assistant, ward assistant, community-care worker, and others. Two hundred and sixty different titles associated with the role were identified in a scoping exercise done in Wales (Health Professions Wales HPW 2004). Without regulation, these titles are not protected unlike the title of "nurse." Consequently anyone can put on a badge that reads "healthcare assistant" or equivalent and no one is any the wiser in terms of how much or how little training that individual has had (Figure 1.1). Regulation should eliminate this scandalous anomaly and would result in standardised training, competencies and conduct for the HCA and a clearer understanding of the role for all concerned, thereby ensuring safer practice and improving the outcome for the worker, the employer and most importantly, the patient. Unfortunately the wheels of bureaucracy grind very slowly and whilst it is recognised by most people that Regulation must be the way forward, it is still a long way off. At present we are still only at the stage where the need

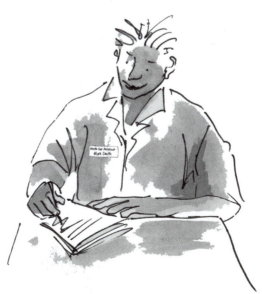

Figure 1.1 Healthcare assistant.

for 'assured voluntary registration' has been recognised (DH 2011a) but there are inherent weaknesses in this approach. Only those who are sufficiently motivated will opt for voluntary registration, and those who do not are more likely to include the ones who are already falling behind in standards of training and care. The RCN supports the statutory regulation of HCAs and Assistant Practitioners (Hand 2011) and identifies that this would be in the interest of improved public safety (RCN 2007; 2009).

The call for regulation has been given a huge boost with the publication of The Francis Report (The Mid Staffordshire NHS Foundation Trust Public Inquiry 2013). The Inquiry was set up following the disclosure of appalling care resulting in patient suffering and in many cases premature death in hospitals within the Mid Staffordshire NHS Foundation Trust.

The report makes many recommendations including the need for a uniform description of healthcare support workers that clearly distinguishes them from registered nurses. It also recommends that healthcare support workers working for the NHS or for the independent sector should be registered and have a National Code of Conduct with a common set of national standards for education and training to be overseen by the Nursing and Midwifery Council.

Until this happens, we should endeavour to promote the idea that HCAs should have the opportunity and be actively encouraged to attend relevant courses and achieve accredited training to ensure competence in their area of work. It should not be acceptable for HCAs to be trained in the workplace when the quality and consistency of training cannot be ensured. The public (you and me!) have a right to expect that when they are treated by a healthcare worker, that person has the relevant training and competence.

Section II
Some Useful Stuff

Understanding Reflective Practice

2

WHAT IS REFLECTION AND WHAT IS THE POINT?

What happens when something goes wrong at work? Suppose, for example, that you take a blood sample but forget to label it; or a patient becomes angry and hostile after being kept waiting; or a colleague is critical of your work; or you are asked to do something which you feel is out of your sphere of competence? The list is endless and I suspect many of you reading this will recognise at least one of the examples given. So what do you do about it when it happens? Mull it over for a while then forget about it until it happens again? Chat about it over a cup of coffee with a friend who is on your side and is very reassuring? Or carry on with your busy clinic and think of it as "one of those things"? Or maybe it stays on your mind for a bit longer, at least until you get home when it gets pushed to the bottom of the priority list competing against collecting the children from school or deciding what to cook for supper. If this is what happens then chances are it wasn't a very useful learning experience, and as a result, it is more likely to happen again.

Alternatively and just as importantly, you will have some very good experiences, such as a clinic that goes particularly well or positive feedback on your work from colleagues or patients. You need to learn from all these various experiences and can only do this if you can establish the factors that contributed to the outcome of that practice. Depending on whether the outcome was good or bad, you can then endeavour to change your practice or try to repeat it in the future.

Sometimes it is also useful to question established and accepted practice to determine if that is actually the best way of doing something and consider if or how it could be improved.

Reflection is the process we can use to look back on our work and although it is usually thought of as a tool to learn from mistakes or poor practice, I hope you will discover that it can be so much more than this.

HOW CAN WE LEARN FROM OUR EXPERIENCES?

This is where a structured reflective process can be a useful tool and one worth developing and nurturing as you hurtle through your busy working life. If you can learn to reflect honestly and thoroughly on your work and experiences, you will ultimately become a safer practitioner, protecting yourself and your patients. Your job satisfaction is likely to improve as well.

Reflective practice can enable us to:

- Study our own decision-making processes
- Be constructively critical of our relationship with our colleagues
- Analyse hesitations and skill and knowledge gaps
- Face problematic and painful episodes
- Identify learning needs. (Bolton 2010)

So reflection is a strategy to develop learning and understanding through experience. It allows the practitioner to understand the experience differently and move on to provide safer practice, less likely to repeat past mistakes. Reflection involves consciously thinking about the experience (as opposed to mulling it over for a few minutes) and actively making decisions. It does not need to be intrusive or time consuming and neither should the potential complexity of the skills involved be viewed as a barrier to the process. It can be as simple or as complicated as you want it to be. Reflection is thought to be a way of bridging the theory practice gap (Bulman and Schutz 2004) and is important to enable us to transfer learning into practice (Chapman and Law 2009).

Writing the reflection down is especially useful and can help the process by allowing the writer to effectively freeze the film, reflect on it, rewind and review a previous scene having reflected upon a later one (Bolton 2010). Jasper (2003) suggests that the process of writing things down enables us to unlock secrets that have puzzled us or learn things about ourselves and those around us. It is a "method of inquiry, of finding out about yourself and your topic" (Bolton 2010). Moreover and when appropriate, written records might then be discussed with a trusted supervisor so that you can share your collective experience to make sense of the challenges encountered.

SO WHAT DO YOU WRITE ABOUT AND HOW DO YOU WRITE IT?

Even for nurses with many years of experience, the process of writing meaningful reflection can still be a daunting task. Part of the problem lies in the fact that at times it can be an uncomfortable experience. You might begin to realise that what happened occurred as a direct result of your action, what you did and how you behaved. Jasper (2003) suggests that this is a very mature way of learning, to be able to revisit and take responsibility for actions and choices, but for this to occur you need to be self-aware and have considerable insight into your behaviour and this can take time to develop. So, writing the reflection down (Figure 2.1) also becomes a way of 'knowing' and a method of discovery and analysis (Bolton 2010).

Compiling a reflective diary is a good starting place for those of you who are new to reflective writing. There are also many frameworks or tools that have been developed to assist in the art of structured written reflection and they may help as a reminder of the different dimensions of reflection and dissuade us from focussing on only that which seems comfortable or convenient. We are all good at telling

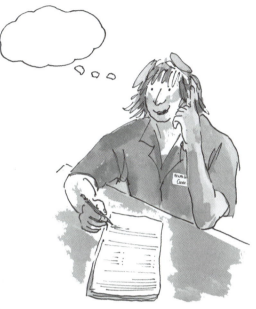

Figure 2.1 Reflection.

stories, but all too often our stories are uncritical and self-protective, providing us with an acceptable explanation of what happened in order to make us feel better about ourselves. Our stories are an attempt to create order out of chaos, but they rarely provide us with the opportunity to develop as people. To do this we need to try and look at the story from a different and maybe strange point of view. We need to reexamine the story from a different perspective. If we cannot do this we risk only ever seeing the world from our own limited view, in line with our own "truth."

SOME FRAMEWORKS FOR REFLECTION

Gibbs' (1988) reflective cycle is one of the older models but nevertheless is still widely used today. **Gibbs** describes six key stages in the reflective process:

1. Description of what happened.
2. Feelings – what were you thinking and feeling?
3. Evaluation – what was good and what was bad about the experience?
4. Analysis – what sense can you make of the situation?
5. Conclusion – what else could you have done?
6. Action plan – what will you do next time?

Driscoll (2007) provides an alternative framework with three simple stages:

1. What? – What happened?
2. So what? – The analysis. How did it make you feel or how do you think the others involved felt and why is it important?
3. Now what? – Action plan. What do you do next?

Oelofsen (2012) provides a three-step process designated as:

1. Curiosity – why do we do things in certain ways, what is my contribution, is there anything for me to learn from my own actions?
2. Looking closer – a journey towards understanding. Taking a closer look at the event to reflect on it according to the questions produced at Step 1. Remember though that there are not always clear answers to questions, but they may provide us with the impetus to find out more.
3. Transformation – a journey towards action, using the understanding gained and starting to implement new ideas. This stage is about enhancing personal competence and improving service.

EXAMPLE OF A REFLECTIVE ACCOUNT

The framework used here is the Driscoll (2007) Framework for Reflection, but any of the many available frameworks could be used with equal effect.

Keeping Patients Waiting – the Dilemma Faced by a Nurse Practitioner

What?

I always run late – it is not so much that I am a poor timekeeper, but has more to do with the fact that my consultation times are not long enough. How can I possibly have an effective consultation in ten minutes? Patients always have more than one problem and I am not very good at saying "No" or suggesting that they rebook for another appointment to discuss other problems. The trouble is that this often this results in patients on the end of the list, waiting up to an hour, as each previous consultation has run over by about five or ten minutes. Some of my GP colleagues have a similar problem, but others are very good at sticking to time. Unfortunately patients who have long lists of problems avoid the doctors who are good timekeepers as they know their own consultation time will be limited, but at least those doctors don't keep their other patients waiting.

So what?

My patients sometimes get angry if they have been kept waiting and this increases my personal stress levels. This problem could be the fault of the system that only allows me ten minutes and doesn't provide enough staff to deal with the numbers of patients. Or it could be the fault of the patient who is too demanding and too impatient. Surely if their problems are that important they should understand and not mind waiting? They need to rearrange their busy lives to fit in with mine, don't they?

But how would I feel as the patient? I was kept waiting all night in a busy A/E department once and it wasn't much fun. I was very uncomfortable and anxious and I was in a little room without windows. I was completely convinced I'd been forgotten about. No one came to tell me what was happening. Why did this strike me as unacceptable when I routinely do this to my patients every day? Is there another way to organise my working day to make this situation easier even if I can't solve it completely? Could some or even most of the fault here actually be mine? I suppose it could and if I'm honest instead of defensive, then it probably is. Why should people wait for me? And why do I always take a long time? Some of this probably stems from the fact that I am very conscientious which is not a bad thing. However, some of it may be due to the fact that as a nurse practitioner, I feel I need to make sure that decisions I make are beyond reproach. I sometimes feel as if I am on trial compared with my doctor colleagues. I feel the need to evoke confidence in my patients and make sure they will be cared for as thoroughly if not more so than if they went to see the doctor.

I need to recognise that it is important to me to have time to spend with my patients, to feel I have given of my best for them. However, this doesn't work if we start off on the wrong foot, with the patient feeling annoyed for having to wait so long and if I am feeling stressed because I know I have kept them waiting.

Now what?

I will discuss changing my appointment system with the practice manager so that I have some catch-up slots in between patients. This may mean that my clinic will finish later than my colleagues', but then it usually does anyway. I will start encouraging my patients to restrict their problems to one per consultation so I don't get swamped. I will research and practice some assertiveness skills to help me with this. I will also make a point of asking the receptionists to inform the patients if I am running late so they have the opportunity to rebook if they cannot wait. I will reevaluate this in one month to see how it's going.

Evaluation at one month

I have now changed my appointment system to allow three ten-minute gaps to catch up, and so my clinic goes on for thirty minutes longer. I recognised the need to manage my consultation time, but I do still struggle with asking a patient to rebook for another appointment when they have more than one problem. I haven't yet addressed my assertiveness skills to help me with this problem, so I will do this by the end of the month. Sometimes I do still run over if I have a patient who needs more time when, for example, they need admission or if they are depressed. When this happens the receptionists have informed the patients who are waiting, and so far only one of them has rebooked. My practice has changed, and I feel less stressed and work more effectively. My patients are not waiting as long and are less stressed and less likely to be hostile.

If I hadn't stopped to reflect on what was happening and just accepted the status quo, I would ultimately have felt used and abused, blaming everyone except myself. My job satisfaction was poor, and my patient care was suffering. It has not been a comfortable process, recognising my own shortcomings. But I also recognise that some of these feelings stem from the need to give patients enough time and my need to do things thoroughly.

I hope you will find reflection useful and that you will continue to use and develop this skill in the future. Throughout the book there will be more opportunities for you to practice some structured reflection. Be sure to have a go!

ACTIVITY

Try and restructure the reflection provided using one of the other frameworks. See if you can work out which bits of the reflection fit under the headings provided by the Oelofsen (2012) and Gibbs (1998).

Now have a go at a reflection yourself using any of the frameworks, whichever one you find the easiest to work with. You can even use a mixture of them as long as you have some structure to your reflection so that you avoid waffling and getting nowhere. Be honest about your feelings and how you think others may have felt. Your reflection can be about anything big or small that happened to you at work – something you still found yourself thinking about at the end of a busy day, but keep it simple to begin with.

Understanding Accountability and Delegation

3

In your role as HCA, you will constantly be asked to accept and perform tasks that have been delegated to you by the registered nurse or doctor. It is vital that you and the person delegating the task to you understand the individual roles in the process of delegation and what exactly each of you is accountable for.

When I first started delivering training for HCAs I had many long, interesting, and sometimes heated discussions with registered nurses who were understandably anxious about being held accountable for the actions of the HCA. Since then, HCAs have become so much a part of the team in most areas that I think nurses are more aware of the issues. It can, however, still be a controversial area with some grey areas which are not always easy to resolve. This chapter will attempt to explore and clarify some of the main issues.

DEFINING ACCOUNTABILITY

When you are accountable you are personally responsible for the outcome or the consequences of your actions. There are various types of accountability:

- **Legal accountability**: this is the obligation of every citizen to obey the laws of the country
- **Professional accountability**: this is the additional obligation of the professional not to abuse trust and to be able to justify professional actions.
- **Prerequisites for accountability:**
  - **Responsibility:** Job description, standards, protocols
  - **Authority:** Appropriate registration, training, qualification

Responsibility and authority require knowledge and the ability to understand the alternatives, reasons, and consequences of a decision.

The NMC (2008) advises that registrants (i.e., registered nurses) have a responsibility to deliver safe and effective care based on the best available evidence or best practice.

If the registrant decides to delegate a task to the HCA then these rules still apply and the decision as to which activities are appropriate to delegate lies solely with the person delegating the work. There is no specific guidance regarding which activities can or cannot be delegated. There are very few activities that are regulated, and these include such things as prescribing drugs and certifying death. This has meant that in some areas HCAs are performing quite complex tasks whilst in others they are not allowed to do much at all. A good example that is still creating much debate in various areas of the UK is that of influenza immunisations. Some local authorities have decided that HCAs should never be allowed to give influenza vaccinations whilst others have embraced it as a task very suitable for competent HCAs providing they have a patient-specific direction in place.

DELEGATION

Questions to consider when a task is delegated to a HCA:

- Is this in the best interests of the patient?
- Does it involve clinical risk, and if so is the risk significant?
- Who has the authority and appropriate clinical knowledge to agree that this task can be delegated?
- Is the person delegating the task competent in it themselves?
- Is the HCA competent in the task to be delegated? Will it impact on the work of others?
- Will it be beneficial to the HCA role, and do they have the capacity to take it on?

Having considered these points and decided to proceed with the delegation there are some basic rules that should be followed to ensure that both the person delegating the task and the HCA are protected and that patient care and safety is not compromised in any way.

Be *clear about the task* to be delegated and have clear *ground rules*. Check that the *job description* includes the new task and make sure there are robust procedures or *protocols* in place. These protocols must be regularly reviewed and should specify *when the HCA should seek further advice*. Be sure there is *appropriate insurance cover* for the new task.

Check that *all members of the team are aware of the new task* and the restrictions. Negotiate time for regular *supervision and support* and ensure there is access to *appropriate education or training* for the new task. This training should ideally involve the completion of *recognised competencies* (such as those outlined in the National Occupational Standards) with *written evidence* and there should be provision made for regular *updates* at appropriate intervals.

There are some useful resources online for induction and as an adjunct to training. The RCN First Steps website (RCN 2013a) is one such resource and is available at: www.rcn.org.uk/firststeps.

Finally any new task should be *evaluated* after a period of time to assess the impact on all concerned.

As yet there is no regulation of HCAs so each case will have to be assessed individually, and some will be more willing and able to take on the various tasks than others.

At the heart of this is the undisputed fact that the registered nurse or the doctor is accountable for the *appropriateness of the delegation.* In some instances, nurses have found themselves in a position where they disagree with a nurse or doctor colleague on the appropriateness of delegation to the HCA. In this case they should make it clear from the outset that they will not be held accountable for the delegation and should put this in writing.

So where do *you* as the HCA, fit in all of this? If you accept a task are you accountable? As a HCA you don't have a professional body such as the Nursing and Midwifery Council in the way that nurses do, but *you are still accountable to yourself, your employer, your delegating nurse, and most importantly to your patient* (Figure 3.1). So if you feel you have been delegated a task for which you have not had appropriate training or whenever you are in any doubt about your competence, you should always say "no" until you have had further advice or clarification.

Suggested answers in Box 3.1.

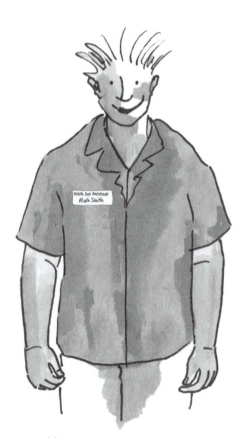

Figure 3.1 Are you accountable?

Case Study: A complicated dressing. Who is accountable?

Now have a look at the scenario presented here and see how you do.

Scenario: A complicated dressing. Who is accountable?

You are working alone as the nurse is off sick, and a patient comes in for a dressing change. The patient has an open wound that requires packing with ribbon gauze to avoid the wound healing over the top too quickly. You have never done this type of dressing before and are not sure you should go ahead and do it, but the patient is insistent as they are unable to get to the local hospital which is twenty-five miles away to have the dressing done, and it really needs doing today. You ring the doctor, and check with him. He is busy with another patient and says you will just have to do the best you can.

What will you do?

If you decide to go ahead, who is accountable if something goes wrong?

Box 3.1. Suggested answers to scenario "A Complicated Dressing"

> You should not agree to do this despite the fact that the doctor has given you permission to do so. You know you are not competent to perform this type of dressing and are not sure that the doctor would know how to do it either. There is no protocol to guide you for this, and there is no care plan in place. You have to be assertive enough to say "no" and find another way of helping instead. Perhaps you could book some transport for the patient to get to the hospital or prepare the equipment for the doctor to do the dressing instead.
>
> If you agree to go ahead and there is a problem afterwards, you will be accountable for accepting a task that you are not competent to do. You could be accused of negligence although ultimately the GP would have to accept vicarious liability for this. Vicarious liability means that the employer, in this instance, the GP, is held liable for the acts or omissions of the employee.

4

A Bit About Protocols

Throughout this book you will see a constant reference to **protocols.** You may wonder what protocols are and why they are so important. This chapter will discuss the issue of protocols in practice and provide some tips on how protocols are prepared. I have used the word *protocol* in the chapter title as this is the term most practitioners are familiar with, but you may also use the term *clinical guidelines,* and the two terms will be used interchangeably.

For HCAs who perform nursing duties that have been delegated by a senior nurse and for the nurses who are delegating the care, there must be clear protocols in place to protect both parties and to ensure good quality care for the patient. Without written protocols in place, the HCA may be unwittingly performing tasks that are inappropriate to their role or competence. They may also be making clinical judgements or decisions which may ultimately result in unsafe practice.

THE PURPOSE OF A PROTOCOL

> Protocol-based care enables NHS staff to put evidence into practice by addressing the key questions of what should be done, when, where and by whom at a local level. It provides a framework for working in multi-disciplinary teams. This standardisation of practice reduces variation in the treatment of patients and improves the quality of care.
>
> *(NHS Institute for Innovation and Improvement 2008)*

Protocols or guidelines exist at a national and local level. At a national level we have guidelines created by the National Institute for Health and Clinical Excellence (NICE) and other healthcare organisations such as the British Heart Foundation, The British Hypertension Society, The Royal College of Nursing, and The British Thoracic Society. At a local level, guidelines can be produced by trusts, at ward level, or within general practice. A nurse or HCA may be working within national and local guidelines. For the purpose of this chapter, we will consider local protocols or guidelines developed in the work setting. They can include the actual procedure but should also include information about who is able to perform the procedure, the training required, the patient group with inclusion and exclusion criteria, materials to be used for the procedure, referral guidelines, review dates and signatures of all the healthcare workers involved. They should always be based on current National guidelines or current available evidence or expert consensus and should usually be reviewed annually. They may be reviewed sooner if the evidence or national guidelines change. The NICE (2004) identifies the main features of good clinical guidelines:

- The purpose and scope are clear.
- Stakeholders are involved in the process.
- Development of the guideline follows a rigorous process.
- It is clear and well presented.
- It can be applied in practice.
- Conflicts of interest have been recorded.

> Remember if a guideline exists and the nurse [or HCA] has failed to follow it, this may be taken into account in a court of law when deciding if the legal duty of care has been breached (Tingle and McHale 2007)

Clinical guidelines or protocols are advisory only and should never be used without assessing the specific patient or situation first. Depending on the patient's condition you may decide it is inappropriate to use the protocol. If for any reason, the protocol is not followed, the full reason for this with information about the alternative course of action that was taken should be documented. **Always refer back to the nurse or doctor if you are unsure about anything**.

For legal purposes a protocol should be underpinned by good quality information backed up with current, robust and objective evidence. In each chapter on clinical skills in this book, the procedure for the task has been provided and is always based on current evidence or national guidelines. You may want to use these in protocols that you develop with your senior nurse but you should also include other information as discussed previously.

Case Study

Jo the HCA (Level 3) was taking a blood pressure measurement. She had no protocol to work to but was very experienced and considered herself to be competent in the task. A patient presented for a blood pressure check, and his blood pressure was 170/102. Jo thought it seemed reasonable to recheck the patient's BP in 1 month. When he returned a month later, his BP was 220/130, and he was admitted to hospital. The GP told Jo she should have referred the patient to him during the initial visit.

In this instance, Jo had made a clinical judgment based on inadequate knowledge and training. She did not have a protocol so she had to make this decision for herself or constantly refer back to the nurse for advice. The protocol for blood pressure monitoring should clearly state the correct procedure, as well as the parameters for action including monitoring intervals and when to refer back to the nurse or GP. This ensures that HCAs are never put in a position where they have to make a clinical decision. In a court of law, Jo could be held accountable for making a decision for which she was not qualified. The nurse who delegated the task could also be held accountable, and both the HCA and the nurse could be accused of negligence. The GP employer would then accept liability under the vicarious liability principle.

Section III
Before You Start:
The Basic Ingredients

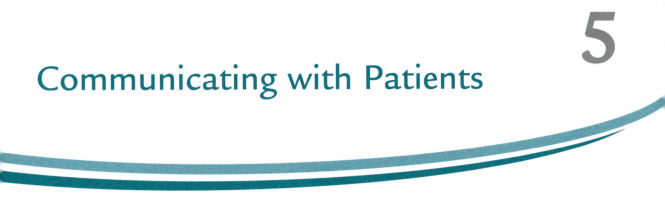

Communicating with Patients

Communication is a huge topic, and there are many very good books available on the subject.

This purpose of this chapter is to raise awareness of the issues around communicating with patients and consider some of the ways by which we can improve our skills to enable us to become more *effective* communicators and thereby improve our patient care.

WHY IS GOOD COMMUNICATION SUCH AN INTEGRAL PART OF EFFECTIVE HEALTHCARE?

There is mounting evidence for the potential benefits of effective communication in healthcare. When the patient understands what is going on and feels that they have been listened to and that they have some element of control over their fate, there are many potential benefits:

- Improved compliance (now usually referred to as concordance) with treatment and improved clinical outcomes (Beach et al. 2006).
- Higher levels of patient satisfaction with fewer complaints. (Clever et al. 2008)
- Better information gathering from the patient.
- Reduction in pain and anxiety (Dougherty and Lister 2007).
- Reduction in unnecessary or inadequate treatment and subsequent reduction in cost.
- Higher levels of job satisfaction for the healthcare worker (McGilton et al. 2006).

What is communication?

I have struggled to find a definition of communication that says or communicates exactly what I feel is important. There are many definitions available for the term in general and some more specific definitions for what it means in the realms of healthcare. Life itself depends on people communicating effectively with each other whether it is verbal or nonverbal and all healthcare must have good communication at its core. When we are with other people we are constantly communicating either by talking, using the tone and volume of our voice as well as the actual words, or through our body language, our gestures and facial expressions. We can also communicate a message or an impression through our choice of clothes and general appearance. (Box 5.1 lists some of the various methods of communication.)

Box 5.1. Methods of communication

Verbal and written:

Talking face to face or on the phone

Tone/volume of voice

Sign language. Lip reading

Text, email, letter, fax

Books, media, information leaflets

Nonverbal:

Active listening - hearing what is being said or not being said

Touching

Body language, gestures, facial expressions

Appearance, dress

Music

Problems may occur when the meaning of the message is lost or misunderstood or maybe never received in the first place.

We all like to think of ourselves as good communicators but may be surprised to discover how often patients take the wrong message away with them. So what are we doing wrong?

The actual *understanding* that takes place is perhaps the single most important factor in communication, so the effectiveness of the communication can be measured by the similarity behind the idea transmitted and the message that has been received. In other words has the receiver, i.e., the other person (or group of people) understood and taken away the message we want to convey?

> The single biggest problem in communication is the illusion that it has taken place.

> *John Powell*

VERBAL COMMUNICATION

When we talk to patients there are several factors to take into consideration:
We must make sure that what we say is:

- Clear: Make sure that what you say is unambiguous so that the patient is left in no doubt about your instructions. Ask the patient if they understand and if they have any questions.
- Accurate: Only ever give advice or information from objective and evidence-based resources. When you don't know something or are unsure about the accuracy of your information, refer the patient to the appropriate health professional.

- Honest: Avoid false reassurance.
- Appropriate to the age and level of understanding of the patient (RCN 2013b).

NONVERBAL COMMUNICATION

How we say something is just as important, if not more so, than *what* we actually say. We have to be aware of the potential effect nonverbal communication may have on our patients. It has been suggested that 93 percent of "emotional meaning" is found in the person's facial expressions and tone of voice, and only 7 percent is from what the person actually says (Borg 2010).

Some points to consider:

Be aware of your facial expressions. Even the most subtle movement in the facial muscles such as a raised eyebrow, can imply surprise or criticism and may make the patient feel uncomfortable because they may feel they are being judged.

Think about body posture. If you fold your arms and cross your legs, this is called closed body posture and will not encourage a patient to open up and talk. But, if you adopt an open body posture or mirror the way your patient is sitting, they will feel more comfortable and talk more freely (Figure 5.1). Try it out on your friends and see what happens!

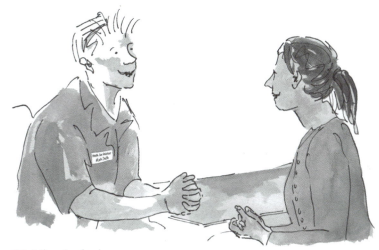

Figure 5.1 Mirroring body posture.

Of course there may be times when closed body posture is necessary, if for example, a patient is very chatty and you need to get on with your work.

Watch your gestures. Pointing a finger can come across as very aggressive or patronising. There are some cultural differences to be aware of too. 'Thumbs up' is not necessarily a friendly gesture and in Greece for example, it may be considered quite rude.

Consider your appearance. What are you communicating to your patients if you turn up at work with your hair untidy and with a dirty uniform on (Figure 5.2)? You might have just been in a rush but the chances are that your patient will conclude that you are uncaring or slapdash in your approach. This is not a good start in a consultation and may not give your patient much confidence and it may not actually convey the type of person you are at all.

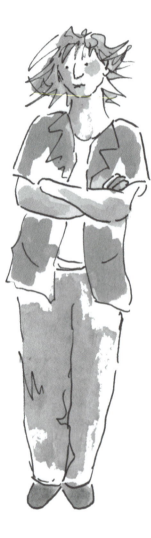

Figure 5.2 Untidy HCA.

Are you a good listener?

Have you ever had a conversation with someone who is *not* a good listener? They just seem to be waiting for you to finish, so that they can make their own comments and they are not actually listening to what you are saying. How does this make you feel? Do you enjoy talking to these people?

Really listening or 'active listening' to what someone is saying and more importantly sometimes, to what they are *not* saying, is a skill that takes practice. It is often difficult to listen properly when you are busy or distracted, but it is well worth it in terms of what you can actually learn about your patient. It also makes them feel that you care about them and that they are valued. Maintain eye contact and avoid the temptation to look at the computer or at your watch while the patient is talking. At intervals during the consultation, reflect and summarise back to the patient what you think they have told you to check that your information is accurate and to show that you have been listening.

"So Mr. Jones, just to clarify, you said you had been feeling unwell for three weeks now and your pain is getting worse?"

OVERCOMING BARRIERS TO COMMUNICATION

There are many barriers to effective communication. Sometimes there is nothing we can do about these but often there are things we can do that will help.

- **Practical difficulties.** For patients with impaired hearing or sight, physical disability or learning difficulties it might be useful to write or type information clearly or in large font. Always face the patient, speak clearly and never shout. There are many resources available for patients with various types of disability. There are leaflets in Braille for the blind, leaflets in different languages and some for patients who may not be able to read that include drawings to explain various clinical procedures.
- **Fear, anxiety, pain and fatigue.** Remember many patients feel vulnerable and alone and when faced with illness. They may appear to be aggressive or may be unable to take in much information if they are frightened or in pain. Be tolerant and understanding and avoid giving more information than necessary until the patient is calmer or feels better. It is our role to try and reduce the patient's anxiety and build their confidence when we can.
- **Interruptions and distractions during the consultation.** Turn the phone to silent and make sure the room is private and free from distraction. Discourage colleagues or patients from knocking on the door when you are with a patient.
- **Using medical terminology.** Talk in a language your patient can understand. Working in the clinical environment we become very used to medical jargon and forget that to our patients it is sometimes like a foreign language. Avoid medical terms and always check that your patient understands what you are talking about.
- **Mismatched agendas.** Is your agenda the same as your patient's? For example you may want them to stop smoking but they may not have any intention of stopping. They may want to discuss their depression when your remit is to record their blood pressure. Try and make sure you are both there for the same purpose or effective communication becomes difficult. (Box 5.2. Case Study: A breakdown in communication.)

- **Clash of personality.** Do some patients get on your nerves or rub you the wrong way? Never mind how hard we try, there will always be some patients we cannot get on with and some that make our heart sink. Keep your attitude professional and calm. Avoid confrontation and check that the pitch of your voice doesn't rise, indicating irritation. Try some of the assertiveness techniques discussed in the next chapter. Alternatively if there is someone you really cannot get on with, you may need to make sure this patient is booked in with someone else if possible.

- **Language and cultural differences.** Lack of communication is more likely to occur when nurses care for international and culturally diverse persons (Ludwick and Silva 2000).

  This can result in misunderstanding and lack of respect for people whose cultural values are different. As care providers we owe it to our patients to be aware of our own cultural values and biases and to be alert to the misunderstandings that may occur as a result.

  If the patient does not speak English you may need to utilise an appropriate resource for interpretation such as "Languageline" available at www.languageline.com.

- **Over familiarity.** We may feel we are just being friendly or trying to relax a patient by using an endearment such as "my love'" or "darling" or by using their first

Box 5.2. Case Study: A breakdown in communication

Jenny the HCA was helping the nurse run the diabetic clinic. She performed the physiological measurements before the patient saw the nurse. She would often overhear the nurse talking to her patients and realised it made her feel quite uncomfortable. On one occasion the nurse appeared to be scolding the patient. She spoke quite loudly and sounded like a teacher addressing a naughty child, reprimanding him for indulging in a high-fat diet. The man sat back and folded his arms and crossed his legs. He was polite but said little throughout the consultation. At the end of the appointment when the patient had left, the nurse sighed and said, "How can we help these patients when they won't help themselves? I feel like I'm banging my head against a brick wall most of the time."

Jenny privately sympathised with the patient, and she wondered how much if anything he had learned or benefited from the appointment.

In this situation, the nurse had created a barrier to effective communication by patronising the patient instead of engaging him as an equal partner in the consultation. It would have been helpful to explore why he chose to eat unhealthily and assess his readiness for change. If he indicated an awareness of his unhealthy diet and a willingness to change, she could then have provided him with the appropriate written information. By adopting an authoritative stance and treating him as if he was stupid, she alienated her patient, and he clearly demonstrated disengagement by his closed body language. The message the nurse intended to send was not received, and communication broke down.

name instead of giving them their full title. However this sort of language may be interpreted by the patient as over familiar or disrespectful. Always ask permission before calling a patient by their first name and avoid the use of endearments. Take care not to invade a patient's body space or touch them inappropriately. You might be very tactile in your personal relationships, but you should keep a distance in professional relationships. Touching someone gently on the arm can be useful to show that you care, but more than this is rarely appropriate.

In summary, communication should be patient centred and responsive to the patient's needs, preferences, beliefs and values. To communicate effectively with patients we should endeavour to:

- Choose the best method to communicate
- Remove the barriers to communication when possible
- Stop to ask questions, clarify, and check understanding
- Listen sincerely and with empathy and warmth
- Consider cultural differences
- Know our audience and respect them

Simple Assertiveness Skills

6

Many HCAs find themselves in a difficult position when they have previously been working as a receptionist or on the administrative team in the same place of work. They are used to doing work for the doctor or nurse often without questioning, based on the supposition that in clinical matters the nurse or doctor knows best. In their new role they have to be able to refuse to accept a task if they feel it is outside their sphere of competence. Some doctors and nurses may not always have a clear idea of what HCAs can and cannot do and may not understand why the HCA might appear reticent to agree to a new task which may seem very simple and straightforward to them. It can also be very flattering when the doctor or nurse has such faith in their HCA and assume they will be more than happy and capable to take on a new role. The HCA might then feel that they are in some way letting down their medical colleagues or disappointing them if they are doubtful about their own ability and refuse to accept a delegated task. They may also find themselves in the same position with reception staff or patients who now see them in a clinical domain and so view them as "a nurse" and therefore assume them capable of advising on complex health issues or checking a wound. The HCA has to develop the ability to say "No" assertively when necessary without being seen as awkward or lazy and without creating confrontation or confusion.

WHAT IS ASSERTIVENESS?

Let's think about what assertiveness is. Maybe you have heard the term directed at somebody who comes across as a bit bossy or over confident. It is a term that is often misused and is even used as a term of abuse at times. This is because it is being confused with aggressiveness but in fact it is quite different and it is essential to understand that difference.

Assertiveness means acting in your own best interests but also respecting the rights and feelings of others. If you are truly assertive you should be able to express positive and negative feelings comfortably without undue anxiety. Aggression, by contrast, usually involves an attempt to dominate others with the aggressor standing up for their own interests at the expense of the rights of others. Aggression ignores or dismisses the needs, wants and opinions of others. It can take many forms including verbal abuse, physical abuse, manipulation, bullying, emotional blackmail, exclusion of others, judgemental attitudes to name but a few.

> The basic difference between being assertive and being aggressive is how our words and behaviour affect the rights and wellbeing of others.
>
> *Sharon Anthony Bower (2004)*

The other end of the scale (Figure 6.1) is when we act *passively*. In this case, we fail to stand up for our rights or doing so ineffectively. We might express our needs or opinions in an apologetic, self- effacing way. We will try and avoid conflict and try to please others. This type of behaviour may be more of a problem for the HCA who is new to the role and anxious to please.

In either case, whether we behave aggressively or passively, the results can be equally harmful to ourselves and those we are interacting with.

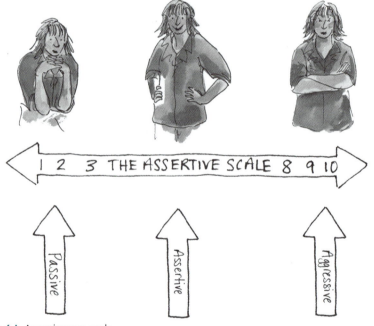

Figure 6.1 Assertiveness scale.

To be truly assertive we must:
- Decide what we want
- Decide if it is fair
- Ask clearly for it
- Not be afraid of taking risks
- Be calm and relaxed
- Express our feelings openly
- Give and take compliments easily
- Give and take fair criticism (Lindenfield 2001)

Saying no

Perhaps the most important thing to learn first is how to say no (Figure 6.2). When a colleague or patient asks you to do something that you feel inadequately prepared for: Notice your gut reaction. If you are in doubt then say so without giving excuses. If you feel unsure then ask for more time to consider the request, but if this latter response is just playing for time when you know your answer should have been no, then don't prevaricate. Say so directly, calmly, without raising your voice.

If saying no puts the requester in a difficult position, think of possible alternatives that you are trained to do that may help. For example, if a doctor asks you to do an injection when you are not competent to do so, refuse politely but offer to fetch the injection for him or her to do it, or offer to make another appointment for the patient to come back for the nurse to do it.

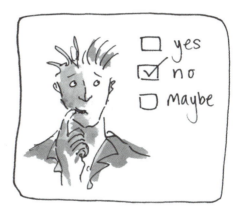

Figure 6.2 Saying 'no'.

Broken record technique (Smith 1975)

This is a useful technique in many different situations, such as responding to coldcallers or salespeople, returning faulty goods, and refusing to take on an inappropriate task

For example if a patient asks you to break confidentiality, how will you say no?

Mrs Brown:	While I'm here can you tell me the results of my husband's blood tests please?
Susan:	I'm not able to give you any information without Mr Brown's consent.
Mrs Brown:	But that's ridiculous – we're married and don't keep any secrets from each other. Please give them to me.
Susan:	There are very clear rules on confidentiality and I cannot break them so I'm not able to give you that information without Mr Brown's consent.

Mrs Brown:	This is quite outrageous - I think I'll have to report you to the Practice Manager unless you give me the results.
Susan:	I am sorry if you're upset about this Mrs Brown but I cannot give you that information. If you would like to speak to the Practice Manager about it then perhaps we can come to some other arrangement with your husband's consent, so that we can give you his results in the future.

The same phrase, maybe with slight alterations or explanation, is repeated in a calm, relaxed manner. Take care to start with the mildest stance only becoming more assertive if necessary. Avoid jumping in with an aggressive or passive stance. If you need time to think the request over then say so. If you practice this technique on the next cold caller you will be amazed at how quickly they give up! But as with all assertiveness techniques you need to practice.

Coping with criticism

One more assertiveness tip that is worth developing is the ability to accept and cope with criticism. This can help you in personal and work relationships.

Accept that the other person has the right to criticise you. Now determine if the criticism is *valid or invalid* (Michel 2008). This is the whole point. If it is valid then accept it and learn from it regardless of how it may have been made. Separate the content (which may be valid) from the way it is given, and don't take it personally. If it is unclear then ask for clarification - 'I'd like you to give me some examples of what you mean'.

Most importantly, if it is invalid or unfair then don't take it on board. Never beat yourself up and allow your self-esteem to be battered by unfair or invalid criticism. You might choose to respond by using an "I" statement, for example, "As I see it . . ." Or you might choose to ignore it, but however you respond, do not allow it to affect you.

There is not enough space in this one chapter to go through all the different ways of developing and improving your assertiveness skills, but I hope this has given you some food for thought. Remember your rights and responsibilities, and keep calm!

There are many good resources online that are worth exploring for more information on how to be assertive, and there is a wealth of books on the subject. Start with a few small changes and build on those. And remember you also have the right to be non-assertive when it suits you as well, as long as this doesn't violate anybody else's rights of course!

ACTIVITY

Now read the following passage and try and answer the questions.

Penny has just taken on the role of HCA having previously worked in reception. She is running a busy blood clinic and notices that she has too many patients squeezed in so that she struggles to get her clinic finished on time for the samples to be collected. Later that day, the laboratory technician rings the

ACTIVITY cont... surgery complaining that the samples have been incorrectly labeled. Over the course of the next month the same thing keeps happening, but Penny does not like confrontation and is reluctant to complain about the situation. She puts her head down and soldiers on and hopes that everyone will notice how hard she works without complaining. She feels terrible because she is constantly rushing and cannot do her job properly. She blames the girls in reception, who she feels must be jealous of her new role and are trying to make life difficult for her.

The laboratory staff have complained three times about incorrect labeling and as a result of this the practice manager asks Penny to explain herself. He criticizes her for not pointing out how busy she was and not attempting to rectify the situation. Now she feels even worse and as if the whole world is against her.

How is Penny behaving? How could she have acted assertively to change this situation?

Suggested answers to activity in Box 6.1.

Box 6.1. Suggested answers to activity

Penny is acting in a passive way in the mistaken belief that people will be pleased with her efforts to cope with the workload. Instead of this, she makes mistakes, and people around her become irritated and annoyed with those mistakes. She is also compromising patient care. As a result she feels unhappy and undervalued.

These are ways she could act assertively:

Arrange a meeting with the practice manager

Print off the overbooked clinic lists as evidence of the problem

Identify how many of the bloods were urgent, and how many could have been booked in a later clinic

Calmly point out that it is not possible to practice safely under this sort of pressure

State calmly and clearly the time required to perform and label a blood test safely

Make an action plan together to address this problem

Document the outcome of the meeting

Evaluate the outcome after a specified period of time

7

Confidentiality, Consent and Record Keeping

CONFIDENTIALITY

As an HCA you will already have some understanding of the importance of confidentiality and of the potential repercussions for you and the patient when confidentiality is broken. Anyone with access to patient information must have a contract that clearly stipulates the principles of confidentiality and the resulting disciplinary action that could result when those principles are not adhered to. This chapter will consider how to maintain confidentiality when dealing with patient information.

WHAT IS CONFIDENTIALITY AND WHY IS IT SO IMPORTANT?

Confidentiality is a fundamental part of professional practice. It is the legal obligation that is derived from statutory and case law as well as forming part of the duty of care to a patient (Beech 2007).

Patients have a right to expect that the information they give to a healthcare professional, will be used only for the purpose for which it was given and will not be disclosed to others without permission (Department of Health 2003). It is important because the patient is in a vulnerable position and depends on the healthcare worker. There has to be trust in this relationship if the patient is to offer vital information and comply with treatment.

Significant legislation has been developed to protect this right (see Box 7.1, Current Legislation).

Disclosure

Disclosure means the giving of information and requires consent from the individual if it is to be lawful and ethical. If possible consent should be freely and fully given. The only exception to this is where there is a risk of significant harm to individuals or groups or society as a whole: examples include child abuse, drug trafficking or serious crime. In situations such as this where there is a need to protect the public interest, disclosure without consent is justified (NMC 2009).

Sometimes information may be shared with other people or organisations not directly involved in the person's care on a "need to know" basis. In this case the

Box 7.1. Current legislation

Data Protection Act (1998–updated 2003) provides a framework to govern the processing of information that may identify living individuals. Personal data should be obtained for specified and lawful purposes only. It must be adequate and relevant, accurate and up to date. It must be protected from loss, damage or destruction and not kept for longer than necessary.

Freedom of Information Act (2000) grants people the rights of access to information that is not covered by the Data Protection Act.

Computer Misuse Act (1990) outlines the requirements for securing computer programmes and data against unauthorised access or alteration. There must be appropriate access for specific staff members only. Shared passwords are unacceptable.

Mental Capacity Act (2005) provides a legal framework to protect and empower people who may lack the capacity to make decisions for themselves.

Access to Health Records Act (1990) establishes the right of access to health records by individuals.

patient must be aware that this information is to be shared unless the healthcare worker feels there may be a violent response. (Box 7.2, Disclosure of Information.)

In some cases, information may be withheld from a patient if the clinician considers that it would cause serious harm to the physical or mental health of the patient or which would breach the confidentiality of another patient.

The Caldicott Report (DoH 1997)

The Caldicott Report was commissioned by the chief medical officer for England when there was concern regarding the increasing use of information technology

Box 7.2. Disclosure Case Study

Susan, the practice nurse, was consulting with Jenny, a patient who was three months pregnant. Jenny had attended for a blood test, but while there, she confided that she was taking amphetamines. Susan was very concerned about the potential risk to the baby and advised the patient against taking such drugs. She documented the consultation carefully but did not explain to the patient that this information would now be available to other healthcare professionals. At a later date when consulting the doctor, Jenny happened to see her notes on a poorly positioned computer screen and was very upset to see what had been written. She complained that this information was confidential, and she had not thought it would be documented. In this case, the nurse was right to document the information because of the potential risk to the unborn child, but she should have made it clear to Jenny that she would have to disclose this information to other healthcare professionals.

resulting in the easy dissemination of patient information. The report outlined several key principles:

- Justify the purpose for collecting the information.
- Do not use patient identifiable information unless necessary.
- Access to patient identifiable information should be on a strict "need to know" basis.
- All health workers who have access to patient information should be aware of their responsibilities and should understand and comply with the law.
- Each organisation should have an appointed "Caldicott Guardian" responsible for ensuring adherence to the above principles.

Avoiding accidental breaches of confidentiality

Never leave records (including those on the computer screen) unattended where they may be read by unauthorised persons.

Never discuss matters relating to patients outside of the clinical setting or discuss a case with a colleague in public where it may be overheard or seen by others from outside the clinical setting such as on social networking sites. Remember that anything you write on social networking sites is never private and can never be completely deleted. There have been well-documented cases of nurses who have made this mistake and lost their jobs as a result. Conduct online and conduct in the real world should be judged in the same way and should be at a similar high standard. Healthcare workers should never put confidential patient information online or post inappropriate comments about patients (Lee and Bacon 2010).

Watch out for accidental breaches of confidentiality. So for example, take care when talking to friends outside of work not to disclose the fact that you saw a mutual acquaintance in the surgery.

Think about telephone confidentiality. Avoid talking to patients on the phone in areas where personal information can be overheard by other patients (NMC 2009). Figure 7.1 depicts an HCA not observing confidentiality.

Always gain the patient's consent before you leave messages on an answering service or with other family members.

Remember if information is passed to another party without consent, the patient may be able to bring a civil claim for breach of confidentiality against the health worker's employer and demand compensation.

CONSENT

Before any examination and before providing any treatment or care, you must obtain consent. You can never assume a patient has given you informed consent just because they are sitting in front of you and appear to be implying that they consent. Do they actually *understand* what the procedure involves, why it is being done, and what the possible benefits, risks, and alternatives are? Do they understand

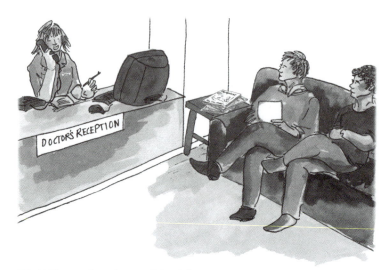

Figure 7.1 HCA not observing confidentiality.

the consequences of not receiving the proposed treatment? If they don't understand the information then they cannot give informed consent. If anything goes wrong following the procedure, you run the risk of being charged with battery (a form of assault) or you may be accused of negligence.

The whole process of establishing consent must be rigorous and transparent (Boxes 7.3 and 7.4, case studies on consent).

Capacity is the term used to denote the ability to use and understand information to make a decision and to be able to communicate that decision.

We assume that every adult has capacity to give informed consent unless the following apply:

- They are unable to take in or retain the information.
- They are unable to understand the information.
- They are unable to use the information to make a decision (NMC 2012).

When giving information about a procedure, it must be given in a way that is understandable to that patient. They must have enough time to consider this information and have the opportunity to ask questions if they want to. We should regard the patient as a partner in the caregiving process and uphold their right to make decisions about the type of care and treatment they receive. We must also respect their decision to decline treatment even if we feel this is not in their best interest. If your patient declines treatment, always refer them back to the nurse or doctor as they may need more detailed information to enable them to make a decision.

Consent must be given freely and never under duress or under influence from the health professional or family or friends. It can be withdrawn at any time during the procedure, in which case the procedure must be stopped immediately.

Make sure that you accurately document discussions that relate to obtaining consent.

Box 7.3. Consent Case Study: Taking blood

Carole the HCA was good at taking blood, but on one occasion the patient developed a large bruise following the procedure. He complained to the practice manager and threatened to seek compensation from the practice for injury. It was discussed as a critical incident, but there was no suggestion that Carole's technique was to blame in this instance. It was recognized that bruising is always a potential complication following venepuncture and may be due to inappropriate activity too soon afterwards as much as to problems during the procedure or poor technique. It was decided that in order to avoid any problems in the future, patients would be given a short information leaflet outlining possible risks including possible bruising and the aftercare required following the procedure to reduce this risk. This would ensure that the patients had the necessary information to be able to give informed consent with an understanding of what was being done and the possible risks. It was also an opportunity to provide written information about the required aftercare to the venepuncture site, advising against heavy lifting or excessive movement within four hours.

This could have resulted in a claim against the surgery because failure to warn of risk is considered as negligence. There is quite a high chance of bruising in this case but the harm is usually minimal. From a legal point of view such a claim would be unlikely to succeed as it is very likely that if told of the risk, the patient would have consented to having the blood test done anyway. Nevertheless it has the potential to create a great deal of stress and anxiety for all involved.

Box 7.4. Consent Case Study: Vaccinations

Margaret was an assistant practitioner and had recently started giving flu vaccinations. This season the vaccination contained three different types of inactivated virus including the swine flu type. On two occasions when Margaret had explained to the patient what the vaccines contained, they had then declined the vaccination as they felt that when they had the swine flu vaccination a few years ago, they had suffered undesirable side effects and did not want to have this problem again. Margaret decided not to offer this information routinely anymore as she felt they were being unnecessarily put off from having it and that it was in their best interests to have the vaccination. A patient then complained when he found out he had received the swine flu type component in the flu vaccination unknowingly and said he had not given consent for this. His complaint was upheld as real consent must be full, free, and reasonably informed, and in this case it obviously was not. The practice was ordered to pay compensation for trespass.

Types of consent

Verbal consent is usually sufficient for tasks that will be performed by the HCA working at Level 3, as described in the introduction to this book.

Written consent is needed where the procedure is lengthy, risky, or complex. This provides evidence of the fact that discussions have taken place and of the patient's decision, but it does not necessarily protect the clinician. If the patient can subsequently prove that they did not have an adequate explanation or they were coerced or rushed into signing the consent form, the consent may be considered invalid.

Who cannot give consent?

Children Under the Age of Sixteen

Legally a person is not considered an adult until they are aged eighteen or over. However, people between the ages of sixteen to eighteen can consent to or refuse medical treatment.

In England and Wales, children under the age of sixteen cannot consent to or refuse treatment as they are considered to lack the capacity, and only the person with parental responsibility can give or refuse consent on their behalf. Sometimes if the child is considered to have significant understanding and intelligence so that they can make an informed decision about their treatment, this rule may be overturned. For contraception and sexual health issues, there is a set of guidelines called the Gillick Competency and Fraser Guidelines (NSPCC 2012), which clearly sets out the criteria required for children under the age of sixteen to be able to consent to their own treatment without the involvement of their parent(s).

In Scotland, the parent's consent cannot override the refusal of a child under the age of sixteen to treatment, when the medical practitioner considers that that child is capable of understanding the nature and potential consequences of the treatment.

> I have had many discussions with HCAs regarding whether it is appropriate for them to be performing procedures such as venepuncture or ear irrigation on children under the age of sixteen. Although this is not specifically related to consent, it is perhaps a good time to mention it. There are no hard and fast rules about this and it will depend on your local protocol and on whether the child will cooperate. Whenever you are in any doubt, always refer back to the nurse or doctor.

People Who Are Mentally Incapacitated (Mental Capacity Act 2005)

Never make assumptions that a person is unable to make decisions or give informed consent, based on their diagnosis, appearance or behaviour. When there is any doubt, the medical practitioner in charge of that person's care should make the decision based on the person's best interests.

No one else can give consent for a person although the medical practitioner will usually involve close relatives to try and determine what the wishes of the person may have been if they previously had capacity, for example where the person has dementia. Sometimes the patient may have made advance decisions on how they wish to be treated if they suffer loss of capacity. They may also choose to appoint another person to make these decisions for them which involves completing a legal form called the HealthCare Power of Attorney.

The Mental Capacity Act (2005) outlines the assessment required to determine if a person is mentally capable of making a decision and the Mental Health Act (1983, amended in 2007) describes the rare circumstances when a patient can be hospitalised or treated against their wishes.

In summary

Consent is an important factor in patient care and you should remember the following key points:

- Always gain consent before carrying out any care or procedure on a patient.
- Make sure that the consent is valid. The patient must have the capacity to consent and you should clearly explain the procedure in a way that the patient can understand including what is being done, why it is being done, and the potential risks and benefits.
- Refer the patient back to the doctor or nurse if the patient refuses or withdraws consent.
- Document that you obtained consent.

RECORD KEEPING

Good documentation is an integral part of care. There is a legal requirement to "do and document" and the law places an equal value on both. Too often we consider documentation to be a chore, but instead we should use it as a tool to transmit and receive information and thereby ensure good quality, safe care for our patients. Good record keeping has a number of important functions.

It promotes:

- High standards of care
- Continuity of care
- Better communication and dissemination of information within the team
- An accurate account of treatment, care planning and delivery
- The ability to detect problems or changes at an early stage
- Clinical audit, research and allocation of resources
- The ability to address legal complaints or legal processes (NMC 2009, RCN 2012b, NHS Professionals 2010).

Remember the quality of your record keeping is a reflection of the standard of care you give and good record keeping usually indicates a safe and skilled practitioner.

Good record keeping – the process

You should record:

1. What you saw or observed beforehand
2. Consent obtained
3. What you did
4. What you saw afterwards
5. The advice that you gave

Record keeping should adhere to the following principles:

- Documentation should be legible.
- Record the event as soon as possible and at least within twenty-four hours.
- The person who made the entry should sign it or enter it under their personal log-in (Figure 7.2).
- Time and date the record as close to the actual time as possible.
- Keep it simple, relevant, and accurate. It should be clear and unambiguous and without jargon.
- Only use abbreviations if they are accepted and understood by everyone.
- Only document facts and not assumptions.
- Involve the patient in the documentation process when possible, so that they are aware of what has been written.
- Record any problems that occurred and the action that was taken to deal with them.
- Never delete or amend records without a full and signed explanation of why this was done (NMC 2009, RCN 2012b, NHS Professionals 2010).

When you record an event, think of the record being scrutinised in a court of law. If this ever happens it probably won't be until a year or two after the event happened. And if it isn't documented, then in the eyes of the law, it never happened!

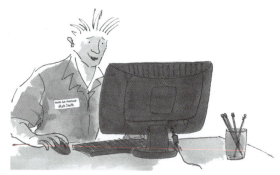

Figure 7.2 HCA on computer.

Health Promotion: The Key Messages

8

As a healthcare assistant you are increasingly at the front line of care and in constant contact with patients from all walks of life who are either healthy or unhealthy or somewhere in between, depending on your and their point of view.

Health is a very subjective thing and hard to define. The best known definition of health is from WHO (1948): "A state of complete physical, mental and social well-being and not merely the absence of disease or infirmity." Some authors feel the use of the word "complete" in this definition makes "health" unachievable for most people in the world (Godlee 2011).

O'Donnell (2009) defines optimal health as "a balance of physical, emotional, social, spiritual and intellectual health' and health promotion as 'the art and science of helping people discover the synergies between their core passions and optimal health, enhancing their motivation to strive for optimal health, and supporting them in changing their lifestyle to move toward a state of optimal health (p. iv)."

As a HCA you are well placed to offer healthy living advice to patients in an attempt to enable them to move towards that state of "optimal health" (assuming that is what *they* want), but you must make sure that the advice is objective and based on current evidence. Use leaflets from objective sources such as NICE guidelines, the British Heart Foundation, Patient.co.uk, and so on. Avoid using leaflets that are endorsed by organisations with products to sell such as some cholesterol-lowering products or those produced by companies such as The Butter Council or The Sugar Council. By giving out such leaflets you are inadvertently condoning the consumption of such products. When you have a uniform on and a badge that says *healthcare assistant*, patients will assume you know what you are talking about. Avoid the temptation to offer them advice if you don't have very good evidence to back up your information.

When offering health advice you should also consider where the patient is on the cycle of change as originally developed by Prochaska and Di Clemente in 1992. It is an old model but still widely used today and most people involved in promoting health are very familiar with it (see Fig. 8.1).

If the patient is in the pre-contemplative stage then "brief intervention advice" is recommended, raising awareness and offering help if required for the future. NICE (2006a) recommends that primary care workers use brief interventions for health promotion advice in areas such as smoking cessation and physical activity. So for example if the patient smokes, ask them how interested they are in quitting. If they

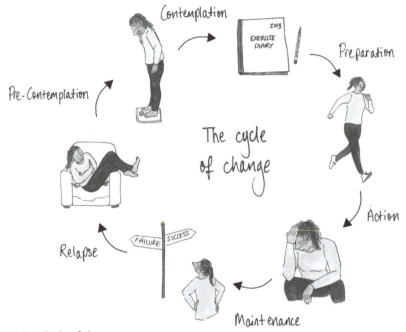

Figure 8.1 Cycle of change.

want to stop, refer them to a support service such as NHS Stop Smoking Services. If they are unwilling to accept a referral, suggest an appointment with a prescriber who may be able to supply them with a stop smoking aid such as nicotine replacement therapy (NICE 2006).

Even 'brief intervention advice' requires a degree of skill and training in health promotion techniques and you should take care not to step out of your area of skill and competence.

As health professionals it is our role to offer advice when a patient wants or needs it. But even when *we* feel they need our advice they still have the right to refuse it. We should aim to empower our patients by giving them the information but remember their right to live their life the way they choose.

If the patient is moving into the contemplation stage or is actually preparing to change, this is when they are most likely to be receptive to healthy living messages.

This chapter will offer some guidance on current messages for healthy living that are evidence based and applicable to most of the adult population. Patients requiring more in depth health promotion for complex problems should be referred to the nurse or doctor or other health worker with training in health promotion.

Key areas for promoting health:

- Healthy eating + alcohol awareness
- Increasing activity levels
- Smoking cessation

HEALTHY EATING + ALCOHOL AWARENESS

There are many well documented benefits of healthy eating (see Box 8.1).

Box 8.1. Benefits of healthy eating

- Lower cholesterol
- Weight control
- Good bowel function
- More energy
- Reduced risk of some chronic diseases, e.g., heart disease, diabetes
- Stronger teeth
- Lower blood pressure
- Clearer skin
- Improved function of the immune system

Most people in the UK are familiar with The Eatwell Plate (NHS Choices 2011a) showing smaller portions of sugary and fatty foods and larger portions of fruit and vegetables and carbohydrates. This is meant to simplify the healthy eating message and demonstrates a well-balanced diet with the emphasis on the "good" foods. Some sources have suggested that sugar should not be represented on the plate at all as it is not necessary in a healthy diet and there is evidence that clearly identifies the detrimental effects of sugar particularly on dental health. One author is pushing the theory that sugar is responsible for the current obesity epidemic (Lustig 2012) and while the theory is worrying, it is, as of yet, unproven. It is certainly a political hot potato and in January 2013 the Labour Party urged the Government to introduce legal limits on the sugar, fat and salt content in food (BBC News 2013).

Tips for healthy eating

This advice is suitable for most people but may vary for groups of people with specific health problems, pregnant women or those with special dietary requirements. They should be referred to the dietician or someone with specialist knowledge if necessary.

Most of the information used in the tips below comes from the Healthy Eating leaflet produced by Patient.co.uk (2012).

1. **Eat plenty of starchy foods** (carbohydrate), such as bread, cereal, pasta, rice, and potatoes. Avoid adding fatty sauces or butter. Use whole-meal products when possible to improve the fibre intake. Avoid cereals that have added sugar.
2. **Eat plenty of vegetables and fruit:** Most people are familiar with the 'Eat 5 portions a day' advice. The portions should be from a variety of sources. Examples of portions are:

   one large fruit such as an apple or pear, banana or orange; one handful of small fruits such as grapes or strawberries; two smaller fruits such as satsumas or

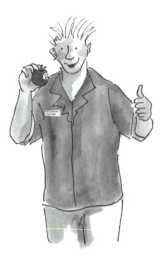

Figure 8.2 Healthy eating!

plums; one tablespoon of dried fruit; one glass of fresh fruit juice (150 ml); three heaped tablespoons of any vegetable.

3. **Eat plenty of fibre:** this is useful to help the bowels function properly and may help reduce cholesterol. It is filling but has few calories. Eating more starchy foods and fruit and vegetables will increase the fibre intake especially if the skin is left on when possible (Figure 8.2). Including pulses such as lentils and beans in the diet will also help to increase the fibre content.

4. **Eat some dairy foods or other calcium rich foods:** Dairy foods are a source of protein and also provide calcium which is needed for healthy bones and teeth. People who don't eat dairy foods can get calcium from calcium-enriched soya milk and some cereals, dark-green leafy vegetables, and tofu. An adequate supply of vitamin D is also needed for the body to be able to synthesise calcium. This can be obtained by exposure to sunlight, but people who are housebound or living in residential homes may need vitamin D supplements.

5. **Eat other protein in moderation:** Foods containing protein include meat, fish, poultry, eggs, nuts, tofu, beans, pulses, and soya. Some of these foods also contain a lot of fat and so should be eaten in moderation. It is widely accepted now that most people eat too much protein although some is important for energy, growth, and repair of cells. It is recommended that the dietary protein comes from a variety of sources especially the lower-fat options such as chicken, fish, lean meat, and tofu. It is also a good idea to include two portions of oily fish per week as the omega-3 fatty acids are thought to protect against heart disease.

6. **Don't eat too much fat:** A low-fat diet may help reduce the chances of heart disease and stroke. It also helps maintain a healthy weight. Reduce the amount of saturated fat such as that found in butter, lard and some margarines. Choose unsaturated fats, such as sunflower oil, olive oil instead. Avoid frying food, choose lean cuts of meat, and watch out for hidden fats in foods such as pastries, cakes and biscuits.

7. **Reduce the amount of sugary foods and drinks:** sugar might make some food taste better and does give an instant burst of energy, but apart from that it is of little value. It can cause weight gain and tooth decay so cutting down on it makes sense.

8. **Reduce the salt:** Too much salt may increase the risk of hypertension and current guidelines advise a maximum of 6 grams a day which is less than that consumed by most people. Try replacing salt with herbs and spices to add flavour and look for foods that contain no added salt. Avoid processed foods, ready-made sauces and packet soups which may be high in salt. Never add salt at the table and limit the amount added in cooking.

9. **Watch the size of portions:** Most people have become accustomed to eating portions that are much larger than required. Try to reduce portion sizes and fill up on more fruit and vegetables. Use a smaller plate and chew food more slowly. Order small portions when eating out. The child size portion is often more than enough for the average adult.

10. **Be alcohol aware:** Alcohol in moderation may be good for us but in excess in can lead to a variety of problems (Box 8.2, Problems related to alcohol). As alcohol has become more readily available in supermarkets with prices much lower compared with those in pubs or restaurants, more people are choosing to drink alcohol at home on a regular basis. This has led to an increase in alcohol related disease and addiction. Alcohol also contains calories.

Box 8.2. Problems related to alcohol

- Liver disease
- Stomach ulcers
- Obesity
- Malnutrition
- Dependence
- Anti-social behaviour, aggression, and violence
- Accidents

Choose healthier non-alcoholic drinks and keep alcohol within recommended limits.

Men should drink no more than 21 units a week and women no more than 14 units and everyone should have at least 2 alcohol-free days a week. For information on units check the NHS website http://www.nhs.uk/Livewell/alcohol/Pages/alcohol-units.aspx.

Also try to drink 6 to 8 glasses of water each day.

11. **Try to sit down at a table when eating:** If you eat in front of the television you are less aware of how much you are eating. Food should be varied, and most of all it should be enjoyed. It is often suggested that the Mediterranean diet is better for us because it contains olive oil, tomatoes and moderate amounts of red wine. Maybe it also has something to do with the fact that it is cooked from fresh ingredients and consumed in company rather than as a solitary activity in front of the television or at a computer.

ACTIVITY

How closely do *you* adhere to the principles of healthy eating? Try keeping a food diary for a week and write down everything you eat and drink. Be honest! Now compare your eating habits with the guidelines given above. Is there room for improvement? How will you make changes to improve your diet?

INCREASING ACTIVITY LEVELS

The World Health Organisation has identified physical inactivity as a major risk factor for heart disease and as a direct cause of approximately 6 percent of deaths globally (WHO 2013). There are many benefits to be gained from exercise and increased levels of activity (Box 8.3). Despite this, self-reported activity levels in the general population are quite low. The Chief Medical Officers for England, Wales, Scotland, and Northern Ireland produced guidelines in 2011 advocating thirty minutes of physical activity on at least five days a week for adults and at least one hour of moderate intensity activity a day for children aged five to eighteen years. (NHS Choices 2011b). Figures published by the British Heart Foundation (2012) show that on average only about a third of people achieved the recommended level of activity.

Tips for increasing activity levels for adults age 19 to 64 years (NHS Choices 2011b) include aiming to be active every day. In addition:

• Over a week, periods of activity should add up to at least 150 minutes of moderate-intensity activity in bouts of ten minutes or more. One way to achieve this would be to do thirty minutes on at least five days a week. Moderate-intensity activities include things that will make you breathe harder and increase your heart rate such as brisk walking or cycling. Alternatively 75 minutes of vigorous-intensity activity spread over the week is equally beneficial. Vigorous activity will make you warmer,

Box 8.3. The benefits of exercise and increased activity

- Lower blood pressure
- Lower cholesterol
- Reduced risk of heart disease and diabetes
- Improved bone density
- Reduces symptoms of depression and anxiety
- Stress relief
- Weight control
- Improved self-image
- Stronger muscles
- More flexible joints
- Greater stamina
- More energy
- Improved immunity

breathe much harder and will make your heart beat rapidly and includes things such as running, swimming, football and skipping (Figure 8.3).

- Include physical activity that will improve muscle strength at least two days a week. Activities to improve muscle strength include things such as exercising with weights, carrying heavy groceries.
- Minimise the amount of time spent sitting for extended periods. Reduce the amount of time watching TV or on the computer. Take regular breaks at work if your job is sedentary.
- Engage in activities that you enjoy and can therefore sustain. Referral to an exercise specialist can lead to longer term changes in physical activity and many exercise referral schemes exist around the country based at local leisure centres. Find out what is available in your locality.

During the writing of this chapter it occurred to me that I had been sitting at the computer for long periods of time so I decided to take my own advice and go for a walk. I walked briskly for thirty minutes and included a steep hill in my walk so I was warm and puffing slightly by the time I got home. I saw my first primrose of the season and felt my cheeks glow as I walked. I must have had a rush of endorphins because I felt so good (and virtuous!) and was definitely reenergized when I sat back down to work. I had also topped up my UV-light exposure and thereby improved my synthesis of vitamin D and absorption of calcium as a result. Who could ask for more?

Try to practice what you preach and you will find it's easier to be more enthusiastic when extolling the virtues of exercise and healthy eating because you know it really works. Patients might be more inclined to take your advice if they can see that you believe in what you say.

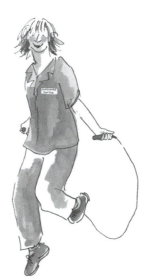

Figure 8.3 Increasing activity levels.

SMOKING CESSATION

Smoking is the single most preventable cause of premature death.

About 100,000 people in the UK die each year because of smoking. The estimated cost to the NHS is £2.7 billion each year. Thirty-four million working days are lost to sickness absence caused by smoking each year. Smokers spend an estimated £2,600 each year on smoking twenty cigarettes a day (ASH 2012).

There are over four thousand chemicals in tobacco smoke, many of which are highly toxic, including things such as acetone, arsenic, benzene, cadmium, carbon monoxide, formaldehyde, and hydrogen cyanide. It is hardly surprising then that smoking is the cause of so much ill health.

Some of the many benefits associated with stopping smoking are listed in Box 8.4.

Box 8.4. The benefits of stopping smoking (NHS Choices 2012)

- Improved sexual function
- Improved fertility
- Younger looking skin
- Whiter teeth
- Better breathing
- Longer life
- Less stress
- Improved smell and taste
- More energy
- Healthier loved ones
- More money

Tips for encouraging people to stop smoking:

Pre contemplation: (Not interested in changing behaviour)
- Accept their position and don't be judgmental
- Check on their long-term plans "Are you planning to continue smoking?"
- Remind them that support is available if they decide to stop

Contemplation: (Thinking about making a change)
- Encourage the patient to talk about the pros and cons and find their own reasons for quitting
- Correct any myths such as 'the damage is done' and remember it is never too late to quit
- Provide information about the local smoking cessation provision

Preparing to change: (Ready to change and be receptive to advice and information)

- Explain that the smoking cessation advisors will support them throughout the process
- Provide a leaflet on Stopping Smoking
- Refer to the doctor for a prescription for nicotine replacement therapy or other medication if appropriate
- Reinforce the reasons they gave for quitting and give praise and encouragement.

Section IV
Core Skills

9

Keeping It Clean – Hand Decontamination

Many thousands of years ago a Greek philosopher and physician named Hippocrates laid down the moral code of conduct for medical practitioners called "The Hippocratic Oath". Within this oath are the words: "All patients have the right to receive care and come to no harm".

As healthcare workers we all have a responsibility to ensure that we uphold this ideal wherever we work. Sadly though, we do not seem to have learnt from past mistakes. This chapter will focus on hand hygiene but remember to think about infection prevention and control in everything you do when dealing with patients. Check your local guidelines for information on dealing with sharps, wearing of personal protective equipment (PPE), and disposal of clinical waste.

SETTING THE SCENE

In the nineteenth century, a Hungarian obstetrician named Ignaz Semmelweis discovered that the likely cause of infection and subsequent death in his obstetric patients, originated from medical students who had performed autopsies resulting in hand contamination. By contrast, patients cared for by the midwives who had not performed autopsies had a much lower rate of infection and death. Semmelweis hypothesised that there must be something on the hands of the medical students that could not be seen but when passed on to the patient, could cause infection. He was able to demonstrate a significant reduction in mortality amongst his patients when medical students washed their hands in chlorinated lime solution. Despite this important finding, his medical colleagues would not believe him. He was later committed to a sanatorium where he died at the age of forty-seven. Twenty years later, Louis Pasteur provided the theoretical explanation or the "germ theory" of disease.

Now many years later, we are still guilty of causing infections in patients because of a lack of basic infection control procedures, the most important of which is hand hygiene.

Healthcare–associated infections (HCAIs) are infections that were not present before admission to hospital or contact with healthcare workers in the community.

The good news is that since a previous survey done in 2006, the rates of MRSA and *Clostridium difficile* have fallen quite dramatically, but other bugs are now emerging and over 6 percent of patients in hospital in England still acquire some form of HCAI (Health Protection Agency 2012).

Each year, 300,000 patients acquire a HCAI in England with 9,000 deaths thought to occur as a result and the cost to the NHS is £1billion a year.

"HCAIs can exacerbate existing or underlying conditions, delay recovery and adversely affect quality of life" (NICE 2012).

The HPA Report (2012) suggests that between 20 to 40 percent of HCAIs may still be preventable and they advise simple measures such as:

- Hand washing
- Use of PPE, such as gloves and aprons
- Regular cleaning to prevent the build-up of organisms
- Isolating patients with specific infections
- Appropriate use of antibiotics and avoidance of overuse

All nurses are responsible for ensuring that risks to patients are kept to a minimum and that their care is as safe and effective as possible (NMC 2008). Good infection control procedures are therefore a priority for all healthcare providers.

WHAT IS INFECTION?

Infection is caused by microorganisms, usually bacteria, viruses or fungi. These are too small to be seen with the naked eye but if fully active and present in sufficient quantity and in the appropriate environment, such microorganisms can become **pathogens** and are then capable of causing infection. All microorganisms are capable of becoming pathogenic. An example of this is a bacterium called *Staphylococcus aureus*. This is one of the major causes of HCAI or community-acquired infection (CAI). Approximately 20 to 30 percent of the population may be long-term carriers of this bacterium. It is frequently found in the nose and on the skin and usually causes no problems. However if the person (or host) has a cut or abrasion, the bacteria can become pathogenic and cause an infection. It can cause pimples, impetigo, or cellulitis. If it gets into the bloodstream it can cause pneumonia, endocarditis, or severe inflammation of the bones (osteomyelitis). Similarly many people may actually have *Methicillin-resistant taphylococcus aureus* (MRSA) bacteria on their skin or in their respiratory tract. When they are healthy and their skin is intact it does not cause a problem. However if they have an open wound or if their immune system is compromised in some way, the MRSA can become pathogenic and cause an infection that is resistant to many types of antibiotics (Patient.co.uk 2010).

Staphylococcus aureus is a very resilient organism but can be removed by correct hand decontamination.

Many different types of microorganisms live on the skin and hands. Some are referred to as **resident flora** and others are called **transient flora**. Resident flora are microorganisms that tend to stay on the skin. They are more difficult to wash off the hands but are less likely to be harmful. Transient flora are microorganisms that are transferred very easily and they tend to be more harmful and more likely to cause infection. They can be transferred by touch from person to person or from person to an object that may then harbour the organism. The good news is that these transient flora are also washed off more easily, so a good hand decontamination technique will remove or destroy them.

Infection prevention and control is not about destroying all microorganisms in the healthcare environment as this is simply not possible. It is about preventing the transfer potentially harmful microorganisms that may compromise the patient's safety and well-being.

How is infection spread?

For an infection to occur the **"chain of infection"** must be unbroken and so the aim of infection control is to break the chain. Good hand hygiene or": hand decontamination" is the most important way of breaking this chain and preventing the transmission of microorganisms

If infection is to occur because of indirect contact via the healthcare workers' hands, the organism must have been present on the skin, it must be capable of surviving on the hands for at least several minutes, hand washing or antisepsis by the healthcare worker must be inadequate or omitted entirely, and the pathogens on

Table 9.1 The chain of infection.

Chain of infection	Example
Source of infection	· Bacteria · Fungus · Virus
Route of transmission	Direct Contact via: Body fluids Or Indirect Contact via: · Hands · Equipment · Arthropods e.g., flies, mosquitos · Airbourne e.g., respiratory droplets
Susceptible host	· Elderly or very young · Immunosuppressed · Open wound/recent surgery · Chronic disease
Point of entry	· Wound · Mouth/nose/eyes/ears · Vagina/rectum

Box 9.1. Five key moments for hand hygiene

When should you decontaminate your hands? The WHO (2009) has defined the key moments when healthcare workers should perform hand hygiene. These include:

1. Before touching a patient

2. Before clean/aseptic procedures

3. After body fluid exposure risk

4. After touching a patient

5. After touching patient surroundings

You may also have included the following:

At the beginning and end of each shift

Before eating

After going to the toilet

After touching your nose

After handling potentially contaminated linen or equipment

Whenever hands are visibly dirty

the caregivers' hands must come into contact with another patient either directly or by being shed into the patient's immediate environment (Teare 2001).

Hand hygiene is the simplest and most important way in which we can reduce the spread of infection and all healthcare workers from cleaners through to consultants have a personal responsibility to undertake adequate hand hygiene.

When Should You Decontaminate Your Hands?

There are many occasions during a day at work when you should decontaminate your hands. How many can you think of? Check your answers against those given in **Box 9.1, Five key moments for hand hygiene.**

HAND WASHING: THE PROCESS

Protocol: use your local infection control policy. You can also download the National Occupational Standard SFHIPC2 *Perform hand hygiene to prevent the spread of infection* to use as a checklist for your competencies (Skills for Health 2011)

1. Remove wristwatches and bangles and any hand jewellery with ridges or stones which can harbour microorganisms, before providing care. When wearing plain rings, such as wedding bands, move them when carrying out hand hygiene, in order to reach all microorganisms.

2. Wear short sleeves or roll up sleeves prior to hand hygiene.

3. Use either liquid soap or approved alcohol-based hand-rub products
4. Hand-washing technique (Figure 9.1):
   - Wet hands under running water before applying soap.
   - Cover all areas of the hands during washing.
   - Rub hands palm to palm.
   - Right palm over the top of the left hand with fingers interlaced and vice versa.
   - Palm to palm with fingers interlaced.
   - Rub the backs of the fingers to the opposing palms with fingers interlocked.
   - Rotational rubbing of left thumb clasped in right palm and vice versa.
   - Rotational rubbing, backwards and forwards with clasped fingers of right hand in left palm and vice versa.
   - Rinse well under running water.
   - When lever taps are not available, turn off the tap using the paper towel.
   - Dry hands thoroughly using soft disposable paper towels.
5. If your hands are not visibly contaminated with organic matter it may be appropriate to use alcohol hand-rub. In this instance, follow the manufacturer's guidelines and make sure all areas of your hands come into contact with the gel using the technique as above for hand washing. Allow the gel to dry naturally before contact with the patient.
6. Keep your fingernails short and clean. Do not use nail polish or artificial fingernails at work.
7. Before each shift, assess your hands for cuts, cracks, and breaks in the skin that could harbour microorganisms.
8. Cover any cuts and abrasions with a waterproof dressing, change the dressing when it appears soiled, and keep the area clean to reduce the risk of infection. Never perform wound dressings when you have a cut or abrasion on your hand.
9. Use hand cream to maintain skin integrity.

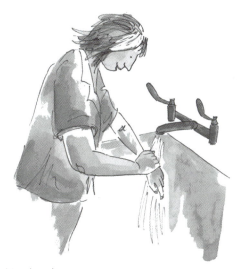

Figure 9.1 HCA washing hands.

10. Report any skin problems to your line manager, or GP so that you can receive appropriate treatment.
11. Report any difficulties with facilities or supplies for hand hygiene to the appropriate person and ask them to take action.

Have a look at the picture in **Figure 9.2.** This indicates the most commonly missed areas after hand washing. Many potentially harmful pathogens could still be present on these hands in the "missed areas." Make sure you never miss these areas when you decontaminate your hands.

LEGISLATION AND GUIDELINES

There are many available guidelines and policy documents relevant to infection prevention and control make sure you are familiar with your local policy as well as some of the national policies and World Health Organization guidelines.

1. Control of substances hazardous to health regulations (COSHH 2002; Health and Safety Executive 2013).

   Under COSHH, all healthcare workers have a legal duty to assess the risk of infection for employees and patients and all others who may be affected by their work. COSHH indicates a possible infection rate of thirty per 100,000 workers per year amongst nurses. Most of these are diarrheal diseases but more serious infections do occur. Four workers are known to have died following needle-stick injuries during work with HIV patients and a further nine nurses are known to be sera-positive because of similar injuries (Health and Safety Executive 2010).
2. National Guidelines for Infection Control (NICE 2012).

   These guidelines provide evidence based advice on best practice for prevention

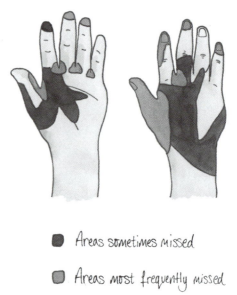

    ⬤ Areas sometimes missed

    ⬤ Areas most frequently missed

Figure 9.2 Areas missed on washed hands.

and control of HCAIs. They identify the standard principles for hand decontamination and the use of PPE, safe use and disposal of sharps and waste disposal. They also provide guidance on the management of long-term catheters and vascular access devices.

3. World Health Organisation guidelines for hand hygiene in healthcare (WHO 2009).

   These guidelines provide healthcare workers, administrators and health authorities with a review of the available evidence on hand hygiene in health-care and makes recommendations regarding how to improve practice and reduce the transmission of pathogenic microorganism to healthcare workers and patients.

Other useful documents

RCN (2012). Wipe it Out. Essential Practice for Infection Prevention and Control
NICE CG 74 Surgical Site Infection (Prevention and treatment).

Now have a go at the activity Box 9.2 Time to reflect.

Box 9.2. Time to reflect

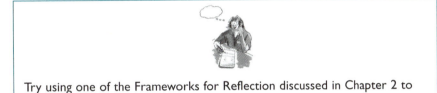

Try using one of the Frameworks for Reflection discussed in Chapter 2 to do this.

We know that hand hygiene is the most important measure for reducing HCAIs but healthcare worker compliance with optimal practices remains low in most settings (Allegranzi and Pittet 2009).

1) During your next shift in work make a note of how many times in the day you decontaminated your hands. If you missed washing or decontaminating after dealing with a patient, why do you think this was?

2) Have a chat with your colleagues and mentor. How many of them decontaminate their hands after every patient encounter or procedure?

3) What would help you and your colleagues adhere to the guidelines more closely?

4) Identify any areas of weakness in your place of work where it is difficult to maintain infection control. Think about things like not having lever taps, no sink in the treatment area, lack of alcohol hand gel, cluttered work surface, etc. Do any of these apply to your place of work? Or maybe you can think of other problems. Discuss this with the other members of the nursing team and identify an action plan to address these problems.

Physiological Measurements

10

Topics to be included:

   Height, weight, and BMI
   Waist measurement
   Pulses
   Respiration
   Pulse oximetry
   Temperature

Whenever performing any physiological measurement always inform the patient fully, explaining what the procedure involves, and make sure that you have consent to proceed.

   Decontaminate your hands before and after patient contact.

   You can download the National Occupational Standard SFHCHS19 *Undertake Routine Clinical Measurements* to use as a check list for your competencies (Skills for Health 2011).

HEIGHT, WEIGHT, BODY MASS INDEX (BMI), AND WAIST MEASUREMENT

BMI = Weight in kg/height in square metres (most computers will calculate this automatically).

Why do we record weight, height, and BMI?
Recording a patient's BMI can be useful for a number of different reasons:

• To identify those people who are overweight or underweight and at increased risk of the associated health problems. (**Box 10.1, Why check the BMI?**)

BMI: Good or bad?

NICE (2006) have produced a classification table to demonstrate the meaning of BMI measurements in relation to a healthy weight and obesity. (See Box 10.2: NICE 2006, Classifying overweight and obesity.)

   While BMI is useful it is not always an accurate indicator of health. The two men in Fig 10.1 have the same BMI but which one do you think has the greatest health risk?

Box 10.1. Why check the BMI?

- To monitor normal growth in children
- To check for abnormal loss of weight, for example in malnutrition, malignancy or alcoholism
- To check for abnormal loss of height, for example in osteoporosis where the spine crumbles
- To enable the doctor to prescribe certain medications or therapies where the dose is dependent on the patient's weight
- To enable accurate measurement of lung function
- To encourage patients who are trying to lose or gain weight

Box 10.2. Clinical Guidance 43, Classifying overweight and obesity (NICE 2006)

Classification	BMI
Healthy weight	18.5–24.9
Overweight	25.0–29.9
Obesity I	30.0–34.9
Obesity II	35.0–39.9
Obesity III	>40.0

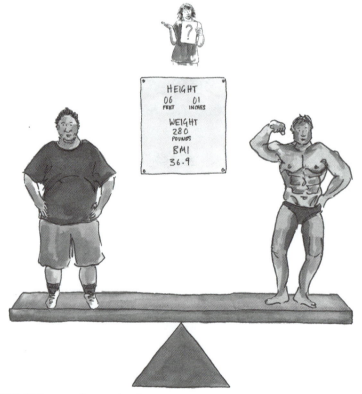

Figure 10.1 BMI – not always what it seems.

Box 10.3. Clinical Guidance 43, Assessing risks from overweight and obesity (NICE 2006)

BMI classification	Waist circumference		
	Low	High	Very high
Overweight	No increased risk	Increased risk	High risk
Obesity I	Increased risk	High risk	Very high risk

For men, waist circumference of less than 94 cm is low, 94–102cm is high and more than 102 cm is very high.
For women, waist circumference of less than 80 cm is low, 80–88 cm is high and more than 88 cm is very high.

Remember that muscle weighs more than fat so if a person is very fit and has built up a lot of muscle, this can render the BMI useless as a determinant of health.

So we need another tool to try and determine if a person is at increased risk of health problems. Measuring the waist in conjunction with the BMI is currently considered to be best practice and is more useful to determine risk. (See Box 10.3, NICE 2006, Assessing the risks from overweight and obesity.)

It is generally accepted that people who lay down fat around their abdomen (the "apple shape") are at greater risk of health problems such as diabetes or heart disease than those people who have a pear shape with larger buttocks and thighs. This is because the type of fat that tends to accumulate around the abdomen appears to block the effect of insulin on the cells, making it harder for the cells to take in glucose. This is thought to create *insulin resistance* so that the body responds by producing more glucose which may eventually result in type 2 diabetes. However, the British Heart Foundation (BHF), in conjunction with the Medical Research Council, have challenged this long held belief and suggest that general obesity may be as important in terms of the adverse effect on heart health (BHF 2011).

Recording height, weight and waist: The process: Protocol!

Measuring the height: Makes sure that the height chart/measure has been attached to the wall at the correct height (Figure 10.2).

Ask the patient to:

1. Remove their shoes
2. Stand upright and look straight ahead
3. Keep heels together and keep heels, calves, buttocks and back in contact with the wall if possible
4. Measure height to the nearest cm.

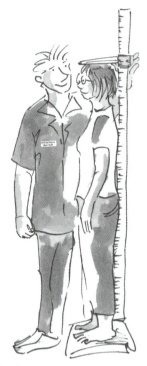

Figure 10.2 HCA measuring height.

Measuring the weight: Use appropriate scales for the task. Recommendations for the types of scales to be used are available online [Local Authority Coordinators of Regulatory Services (LACORS) 2007] (Box 10.4, Inaccurate weighing).

Make sure the scales have been calibrated within the last year (or in line with local policy), are on a hard surface, and are set to zero. Ask the patient to:

1. Remove outer clothing and shoes
2. Stand squarely on the scales
3. Record the weight to the nearest 0.5 kg.

Did you know?

Measurements on analogue scales can be increased by as much as 10 to 12 percent if the scales are on a soft carpeted surface? Digital scales are less prone to this effect (Pendergast 2002).

Box 10.4. Risks associated with inaccurate weight measurement

> LACORS (2007) found that one hospital had used ordinary bathroom scales to weigh a girl with cancer to gauge how much radiation treatment she should receive.
>
> The scales showed incorrectly that the four-year-old had gained weight. Had the inaccurate reading been used, she could have been exposed to a potentially harmful dose of radiation.

Measuring the waist:

1. Use a suitable measuring tape that is designed for the purpose, measure directly over skin or over only one item of light clothing (Figure 10.3).
2. Ask the patient to breathe out normally.
3. Hold the tape snugly (without compressing the skin) around the waist halfway between the lowest rib and the top of the hipbone (roughly in line with or slightly above the belly button).

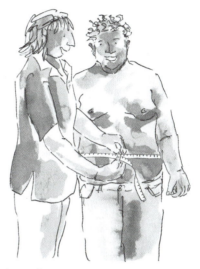

Figure 10.3 HCA measuring waist.

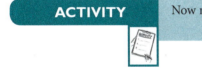

ACTIVITY   Now measure your own waist: how do you score on the Risk Table?

(Box 10.3, Assessing the risk using BMI and waist circumference.)

PULSE RATE

When the heart contracts it pushes blood out through the elastic walled arteries. This is felt at various points of the body as a **pulse**; if the arteries are in good condition, the pulse should usually be felt at the same time as the heartbeat. The normal pulse rate is between sixty to eighty beats per minute but can vary enormously from as low as forty during sleep up to two hundred and twenty or more with strenuous exercise.

An arrhythmia is an abnormal rate or rhythm of the heartbeat. Some are more serious than others. Some are intermittent, and some will become permanent unless treated.

What can affect the pulse?

It may be *higher* than normal (tachycardia = heart rate above 100bpm)

Tachycardia can be classified as sinus, ventricular or supraventricular and there will be different causes for each type. It can occur:

- If there is infection or a high temperature (pyrexia)
- When the patient is anxious
- After exercise
- After stimulants such as coffee or smoking a cigarette
- In some medical conditions, such as hyperthyroidism
- With some medication, for example: adrenaline, salbutamol

It may also be **lower** than normal (*bradycardia = heart rate below 50 bpm*), and this may occur in:

- Athletes
- Some medical conditions such as hypothyroidism, myocardial infarction, pericardial tamponade, adrenal insufficiency, sick sinus syndrome
- With some medication such as beta blockers, digoxin, calcium channel blockers, amiodarone, clonidine, verapamil
- Hypoxia
- Hypothermia

Or it may be **irregular**, without normal rhythm. This can occur in normal, healthy hearts but may also occur:

- In some types of heart disease, for example atrial fibrillation
- Where there is an electrolyte imbalance
- If there are changes in heart muscle
- If there is injury from a myocardial infarction (heart attack)

Pulse amplitude refers to the strength of the pulse and the elasticity of the artery wall. A pulse may be described as strong or "bounding," which may indicate infection.

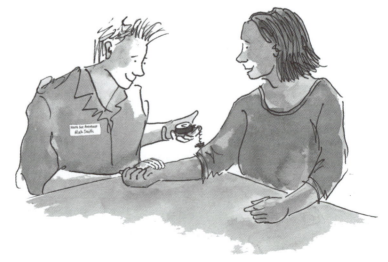

Figure 10.4 HCA measuring pulse.

Or it may be weak, faint, or thready, which may signify shock or hypovolaemia (low fluid levels)

Recording the radial or brachial pulse: The process

1. Use two fingers and press quite firmly over the area at the base of the thumb for the radial pulse and on the inside of the elbow for the brachial pulse (Figures 10.5 and 10.6).

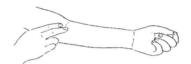

Figure 10.5 Brachial pulse.

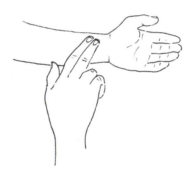

Figure 10.6 Radial pulse.

2. Record the rate by counting how many beats there are in thirty seconds then multiply this figure by two to record the beats per minute.
3. If the pulse is irregular, you will need to measure it for a full minute.
4. Document the result immediately and always refer back to the doctor or nurse if the pulse seems very fast or slow or is irregular. You may also notice if the pulse seems unusually weak or is very strong or bounding in nature. These may be important observations so always report them. (Protocol)

ACTIVITY

Have a look at the body outline in Fig. 10.7 and mark in pencil where you think the different pulse points are. Check your answers on the following page. Using the diagrams in Fig 10.5 and Fig 10.6 for guidance, see if you can you find your own pulses in the wrist (radial pulse) and inside the elbow (brachial pulse).

Measuring a pulse with a Doppler can be useful in patients who have or are at risk of arterial disease, but specific training is required to use the Doppler correctly.

RESPIRATORY RATE

The respiratory rate is a key vital sign, and it is used to detect early changes when monitoring very ill patients.

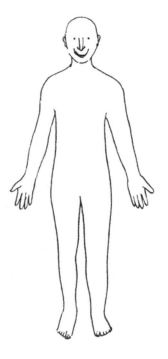

Figure 10.7 Body outline.

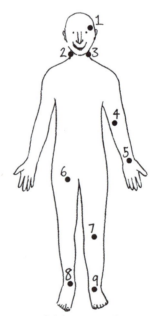

Figure 10.8 Pulse points. 1. Superficial Temporal 2. Carotid 3. Carotid 4. Brachial 5. Radial 6. Femoral 7. Popliteal (behind the knee) 8. Posterior Tibial (behind the medial malleolus or ankle bone) 9. Dorsalis Pedis.

We breathe in oxygen (for the production of energy) and breathe out carbon dioxide (a waste product of metabolism) and most of us will breathe at a rate of about twelve to twenty breaths per minute. It is an essential but subconscious mechanism, and we only become aware of it when it becomes difficult or if we know we are being observed.

The respiratory rate may be affected by:

- Exercise
- Stress and emotion
- Illness
- Some medication

A rate of less than twelve breaths per minute or more than twenty five breaths per minute is considered abnormal (in adults).

Recording the respiratory rate: The process

1. **Look.** Is the patient distressed? Can they complete a sentence without stopping for breath?

   Are there any signs of cyanosis (for example a blue colour around the lips)? Whenever you are unsure always refer the patient back to the doctor or nurse.

2. **Note *how* the patient breathes as well as the rate.** A person who has difficulty breathing will be using all their accessory muscles, sometimes lifting their shoulders up and down in an effort to make the lungs expand. There may be intercostal recession or sucking in of the skin between the ribs and this is one of the key signs of respiratory distress. Some patients will also breathe out through pursed lips. This is very typical of patients with Chronic Obstructive Pulmonary Disease (COPD) and is a method of trying to expel all the carbon dioxide slowly. Rapid expiration is more likely to force the diseased airways to collapse.

3. **Listen to the breathing.** Is there an audible wheeze or other abnormal noise?

4. **Recording a patient's respiratory rate can be difficult because the rate will change if the patient knows they are being observed.** Because of this it is better to count the breaths per minute when holding the wrist as if still checking the pulse rate so that the patient is unaware. As with measuring the pulse, you should count for thirty seconds and multiply by two to achieve the rate per minute. If the patient is breathing irregularly you will need to count for a full minute.

PULSE OXIMETRY

A pulse oximeter provides a non-invasive method of measuring the oxygenation of a patient's blood. It works by shining an infrared light through the tissues of the body and detecting the colour difference between oxygenated and un-oxygenated blood.

A beam of infrared light is passed through the chosen area and the degree of absorption will depend on the amount of oxygen in the blood. Pulse oximeters will often give a reading of the pulse rate as well.

Pulse oximetry is used routinely in intensive care, operating theatres and recovery rooms.

It may be used in a doctor's surgery to monitor a patient's oxygen levels when they are having respiratory difficulty such as during an asthma attack or worsening COPD or during a heart attack. Some patients who are receiving medication that may depress their respiration, such as strong opiate analgesics, may also need to have their oxygen levels monitored.

Accuracy can be affected by the thickness and temperature of the skin, so it is important to place the sensor in the best possible place. This will normally be on an area where the skin is relatively thin such as the fingertip or ear lobe. Other factors such as nail varnish, dirt, foreign objects or bright lighting can affect the light transmission and therefore give erroneous results. Pulse detection may be affected by excessive movement, shivering, poor circulation, and atrial fibrillation.

The normal level for oxygen saturation of the blood is between 96 to 100 percent. Levels below 90 percent can be life-threatening.

Recording pulse oximetry: The process

1. Ensure the patient is comfortable and warm enough.
2. Select a suitable site such as the fingertip, and make sure that any nail varnish, dirt, etc. has been removed. Choose a finger where the skin is not calloused or thickened.
3. Place the probe according to the manufacturer's instructions.
4. Make sure the sensor is also detecting the pulse.
5. Make a note of the oxygen level and remove the probe.
6. Clean and store the probe according to manufacturer's instructions.
7. Document the reading and report any abnormal oxygen levels.

Temperature

Words you need to know:

Apyrexial: Normal temperature – usually considered to be a range anywhere between 36.2°C to 37.7°C.

Pyrexia: High temperature – may also be referred to as a fever, less commonly referred to as hyperthermia.

Hypothermia: Low temperature. We feel cold if our core temperature is 36°C, start to shiver at 35°C, become clumsy and confused at 34°C, develop muscle stiffness at 32°C, and at 28°C would be at risk of cardiac arrest.

The temperature may be taken to check for an infection anywhere in the body when a patient is feeling unwell. It will also be checked routinely post operatively to make sure a patient is not developing an infection. Patients with surgical wounds are more susceptible to infection that can then delay healing.

When you consider the potential implications of an infection for any person, the importance of measuring the temperature accurately cannot be over emphasized. There are various devices for checking temperature but the one used most commonly (and often incorrectly) is the tympanic thermometer. These use an infrared light to detect the temperature at the tympanic membrane (ear drum).

Recording the temperature: The process

1. Place a disposable cap over the nozzle of the thermometer.
2. Press the button to turn it on and then place the nozzle just inside the ear canal and point it forwards.
3. Depress the button until a beep is heard then gently withdraw the nozzle and note the temperature displayed.
4. Remember the device must be placed just inside the ear canal pointing towards the tympanic membrane to take an accurate reading.
5. Always check the manufacturer's instructions for use as the devices may vary slightly.
6. Report any temperature that falls outside the normal parameters to the doctor or nurse.

Other devices may be used in some settings:

7. A rectal thermometer provides the most reliable core temperature but is obviously the most invasive and least "user friendly"!
8. Oral digital thermometers that can be placed inside the cheek (buccal) or under the tongue (sublingual) can be used but must be held in place for long enough and will give a reading that is slightly lower than core body temperature.
9. Body surface thermometers are placed in the axilla or groin but again will need to be held there for long enough and may give a significantly lower result than the actual core body temperature.
10. Forehead thermometers are the least intrusive and can be useful for babies and toddlers.

Now try the quiz below – you can check back in the text for the answers.

PHYSIOLOGICAL MEASUREMENTS QUIZ

1) How do you calculate the BMI?
2) When does the BMI indicate a person is overweight?
3) Why is it useful to measure the waist as well as the BMI?
4) If a woman is overweight according to her BMI and her waist measurement is 78 cm, is she at increased risk of health problems or not?
5) What is the normal pulse rate for an adult?
6) Where would you find the brachial pulse?
7) What is the normal respiratory rate for an adult?
8) List two factors that can affect the accuracy of the pulse oximetry reading.

9) What is the normal level for oxygen saturation of the blood?

10) What is the normal range for body temperature?

 Using a framework for reflection (see Chapter 2), try reflecting on a consultation when you performed a physiological measurement. How did it go, and what have you learned?

11

Understanding Blood Pressure and Performing Accurate Measurements

Measuring and recording the blood pressure is an important task that is often delegate to the HCA. Before you learn how to perform this task it is essential that you understand *what* you are doing and *why*. Only then can you learn how to make an accurate measurement and understand why it is so important.

WHAT IS BLOOD PRESSURE?

Arteries are the blood vessels that carry blood away from the heart. Every time the heart contracts it squeezes blood through the arteries and the blood exerts a force on the artery walls. This force is the **blood pressure**.

Human blood pressure was first recorded in 1847 by Carl Ludwig who inserted a catheter into a patient's artery and connected the catheter to an invention called a kymograph. In 1896 the mercury filled sphygmomanometer was developed by Scipione Riva-Rocci and blood pressure was measured according to how high the pressure could lift a column of mercury (Welch Allyn 2008). We still refer to the measurement in millimetres of mercury (known by its chemical symbol of Hg).

The **systolic pressure** measures the force exerted by the blood on the artery walls at the peak of the left ventricular contraction. The left ventricle is the largest chamber in the heart. (Refer to the chapter on the ECG for more detail of the heart's anatomy.) The systolic pressure is the higher of the two readings.

The **diastolic pressure** measures the force exerted on the artery walls when the heart is relaxed.

The pressure in the arteries will depend on how *hard the heart is pumping* and how much *resistance* there is in the arteries.

There are several things that will create an increase in the resistance in the artery

- If the diameter of the artery is reduced as for example in atherosclerosis where there are fatty deposits sticking to the artery walls.
- If the walls of the artery are stiff or rigid. Think of an old hosepipe compared with a new one. In the new piece of hose, the walls are more elastic and stretchy. The pressure can be absorbed as the wall stretches whereas in the rigid hose the pressure will be greater. As arteries age they become stiffer so blood pressure will invariably increase a little with age.

> The word *diastolic* sounds more relaxed than *systolic* – this is a good way to remember the difference.

- If the blood is thicker or stickier than normal. This can happen when the number of red blood cells increases in a condition called polycythaemia. Red blood cells carry oxygen so patients who have problems taking on enough oxygen (such as those with respiratory disease) may adapt by producing more red blood cells. Smokers may also have this problem.
- If the volume of blood is increased. Again imagine what happens when you turn up the tap and force more water through a hose. The volume of blood may be increased in patients who are having intravenous fluids or those who are retaining fluid such as in kidney disease.

WHAT IS HYPERTENSION, AND WHY DOES IT MATTER?

There are two types of hypertension:

- Essential hypertension where the cause is not known
- Secondary hypertension which may be due to medication (e.g. combined contraceptive pill, steroids), kidney disease or hormone problems.

A patient may be diagnosed with hypertension if the blood pressure measurements show an isolated high systolic pressure (e.g., 180/70), or an isolated high diastolic pressure (e.g.; 130/100) or both (e.g., 170/110). Historically the diastolic reading was considered the most important, but current evidence indicates that the systolic measurement is more important in terms of the potential risk to health (Williams et al. 2008).

In 2003 The Joint National Committee on Prevention, Detection, Evaluation and Treatment of High Blood Pressure used the evidence from a large number of sources to conclude that in people over the age of fifty, a high systolic reading of 140 mm Hg or more is a more important risk factor for cardiovascular disease than a high diastolic reading (National Heart Lung and Blood Institute 2003).

Hypertension can only be diagnosed after several readings (usually a minimum of three) at different times of the day when the patient is relaxed. The phenomenon of white coat hypertension is well known and refers to how some people will always have a higher blood pressure when they are in a clinical setting, probably due to anxiety (often without the patient realising). Recent research has highlighted the problems associated with white collar hypertension, and this has had an impact on the current guidelines that now suggest that all patients should be offered ambulatory blood pressure monitoring (ABPM) or home blood pressure monitoring (HBPM) if they cannot tolerate ABPM (NICE 2011a).

These patients will need to have a twenty-four hour monitor to make an accurate diagnosis or may be advised to purchase a home monitor to perform serial readings at home. In this case they must be advised to buy a monitor that is validated by the British Hypertension Society (BHS) or British Heart Foundation (BHF) to ensure accuracy.

Box 11.1. Websites for lists of recommended blood pressure monitors for use in the home and for clinical use (British Hypertension Society 2012)

> A list of Blood Pressure Monitors validated for home use is available at:
> http://www.bhsoc.org/index.php?cID=246
>
> A list of Blood Pressure Monitors validated for clinical use is available at:
> http://www.bhsoc.org//index.php?cID=247

(Box 11.1 gives the websites where you can download a list of monitors recommended for use in the clinic and in the home.)

The home monitor should be checked against the surgery monitor.

There are various grades of hypertension:

Grade 1(mild hypertension): 140-159/90-99

Grade 2 (moderate hypertension): 160-179/100-109

Grade 3 (severe hypertension): Greater than or equal to 180/110

Do you know when to bring a patient back for further readings and when to refer them to the nurse or doctor? For HCAs who work in primary care, a flowchart based on the NICE 2011 guidelines has been provided **(Box 11.2),** but you may wish to discuss this with your nurse or doctor and amend it in line with your Surgery Protocol.

Box 11.2. Guidelines for HCAs for the referral of patients according to BP

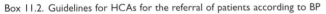

> 180 > 110	160–179 100–109	140–159 90–99	135–139 85–89	< 135 < 85
Refer to doctor on the same day	Recheck three times over next two weeks then make an appointment with the doctor	Reassess three times weekly then make an appointment with the doctor	Lifestyle advice, reassess annually if not on treatment or in six months on treatment	Lifestyle advice, reassess in five years if not on treatment or in six months on treatment

ALL PATIENTS WHOSE BP IS EQUAL TO / ABOVE 140/90 SHOULD BE OFFERED AMBULATORY BLOOD PRESSURE MONITORING - ABPM (OR HOME BLOOD PRESSURE MONITORING - HBPM, IF ABPM IS DECLINED OR NOT TOLERATED).

NICE - CG127 (2011a)

CLINICAL MANAGEMENT OF PRIMARY HYPERTENSION IN ADULTS

How many factors can you think of that might increase your risk of developing high blood pressure and heart disease? Check your answers against those given in Box 11.3

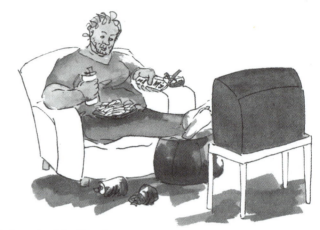

Figure 11.1 An unhealthy lifestyle.

SO WHAT'S ALL THE FUSS ABOUT?

Hypertension is often referred to as 'the silent killer' because usually it has no symptoms, but over time if left untreated it can cause strain on the heart and the arteries. It is one of the most important preventable causes of premature heart disease and death in the UK (NICE 2011). There are many possible complications including angina, heart attacks, heart failure, stroke, peripheral vascular disease, kidney damage, and eye damage. It is often under diagnosed and often inadequately treated.

The role of the HCA in measuring and recording BP *accurately* is therefore vital. When a diagnosis is finally made, it has huge implications for the patient and the NHS.

- There is no cure, and patients will need lifelong treatment.
- It is often best controlled by using two or more medications.
- Many treatments cause side effects.
- More tablets mean more potential interactions with other medications.
- There is increased cost to the individual and the NHS.
- Patients require regular monitoring and blood tests.

Auscultatory or manual method for checking the BP. What are you listening to?

Although many surgeries and wards have now disposed of mercury sphygmomanometers in line with European regulations on mercury control, blood pressure is still recorded in mm/Hg. Many hospital wards and surgeries now use automatic monitors but these cannot be used in patients who have an irregular heartbeat such as in atrial fibrillation. It is therefore important that all HCAs have the training to enable them to take a blood pressure using the auscultatory (listening) method. To do this, the cuff is wrapped around the upper arm and inflated until it compresses the brachial artery. The blood cannot flow through so no sounds are heard through the stethoscope which is placed over the artery. Gradually the cuff is deflated until the blood can just force its way through the artery each time the heart contracts and pushes the blood out. This opening and closing of the artery causes a tapping sound that can be heard through the stethoscope and this is the systolic pressure. As the cuff is deflated still further the artery is open and blood flows more easily so that the forced tapping sound muffles or disappears altogether. This change in the sound represents the diastolic pressure when the heart is relaxed. These sounds are called the Korotkoff sounds after the man who discovered them, and there are five possible sounds that can be detected. You usually listen for **Korotkoff I** when the tapping sound begins to denote the systolic pressure and then for **Korotkoff V** when the sound disappears completely to denote the diastolic pressure. Sometimes the tapping sound may continue in which case you record **Korotkoff IV** – the point at which the tapping sound becomes muffled.

Box 11.3. Risk factors for developing high blood pressure and heart disease

- Poor diet high in fat or salt
- High cholesterol, high LDL,
- high triglycerides, low HDL
- Atheromatous arteries
- Male gender
- High levels of alcohol
- Obesity
- Lack of exercise
- Increasing age
- Diabetes
- Ethnic group
- Family history
- Smoking (although links with sustained hypertension have yet to be established)

MEASURING BLOOD PRESSURE: THE PROCESS: PROTOCOL!

You can download the National Occupational Standard SFHCHS19 *Undertake Routine Clinical Measurements* to use as a check list for your competencies (Skills for Health 2011).

1. Explain what you are doing to your patient and why. Make sure you have their informed consent before you continue.
2. Wash or decontaminate your hands before and after the procedure.
3. Make sure the patient is seated comfortably (preferably sitting quietly for 5 minutes before proceeding). The arm should be free of any constrictive clothing and supported at the level of the heart.

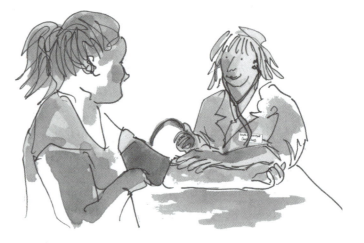

4. Wrap the cuff around the upper arm with the centre of the bladder located over the brachial artery. The cuff must be large enough so that the bladder circles 80 percent of the arm. In larger patients a larger cuff must be used to avoid the risk of inaccurate high readings.
5. Some teaching resources advocate the idea of positioning the cuff so that the tubing comes from the top to avoid noise from the tubing bumping against the stethoscope, being confused with the arterial sounds.
6. It is good practice to palpate the brachial or radial pulse and inflate the cuff until the pulse disappears. Note the readings when the pulse disappears and add thirty. Remember this reading. Now deflate the cuff.
7. Position the stethoscope over the brachial artery and re-inflate the cuff to the level you noted previously. You should not be able to hear the tapping from the brachial artery. If you can still hear it, inflate the cuff a little more until it disappears.
8. Deflate the cuff very slowly (this takes practice). You should record the reading when you first hear the pulse come back in. This is the systolic reading (Korotkoff 1). This should be recorded to the nearest 2 mm and never rounded up or down.
9. Keep deflating the cuff very slowly until the tapping sound disappears or becomes muffled (Korotkoff IV or V). This is the second (diastolic) reading.
10. Measure the BP in both arms initially and record the highest reading. Always use this arm in the future. If the difference in readings between the arms is 20 mm Hg or more, always report this to the nurse or doctor. It may indicate a problem called subclavian stenosis and should prompt further investigation.

11. Take a second measurement from the chosen arm during the consultation. If this is very different from the first reading then take a third reading. Record the lower of the last two measurements as the clinic reading.

12. Elderly and diabetic patients may need to have the blood pressure checked again after two minutes standing to check for postural hypotension (a common cause of falls in the elderly). In this case you should still try and support the arm at the level of the heart so there is no muscular contraction in the arm as this may interfere with the reading.

13. If using digital/automatic monitors, wrap the cuff around the upper arm as instructed in the monitor guidelines. Make sure the arm is free of restrictive clothing and is supported comfortably at the level of the heart. Press the record button and wait for the cuff to inflate and deflate before making a note of the recording. If the monitor indicates an ERROR (e.g., if the patient has an arrythmia) the manual method must be used and the nurse or doctor informed.

14. Always discourage the patient from talking during the procedure.

15. Report the readings or recall the patient for further measurements according to your protocol.

16. BP readings must always be recorded using the appropriate Read Code or template so that they can be easily accessed for future consultations and for audit purposes.

Now try the quiz below – you can check back in the text if you've forgotten some of the answers.

BLOOD PRESSURE QUIZ

1) What is systolic pressure?
2) List two things that might increase the resistance in the arteries resulting in a higher blood pressure.
3) Which artery do you place the stethoscope over to listen for the Korotkoff sounds when performing a manual blood pressure measurement?
4) What is considered to be a normal blood pressure?
5) How many readings are required before hypertension can be diagnosed?
6) If a patient had a blood pressure of 162/98 what would you do?
7) If a patient had blood pressure of 160/110 what would you do?
8) List three complications of hypertension.
9) Which arm should you use to check the blood pressure?
10) What should be offered to the patient whose blood pressure measured in the surgery is equal to or above 140/90 and why?

Using a framework for reflection (see Chapter 2), try reflecting on a consultation where you performed a blood pressure measurement. How did it go, and what did you learn?

Understanding the Heart and Performing the Electrocardiograph (ECG)

12

HISTORY OF THE ECG

In the nineteenth century it became clear that the heart generated electricity. In 1924, Willem Einthoven discovered the electrocardiographic features of the heart and realised that these could be used to detect abnormalities. He assigned letters PQRST to the various deflections and was awarded the Nobel Prize for his discovery.

Before you can understand an ECG or how to perform the test accurately, you need to have a basic understanding of the heart and how it works.

WHAT DOES THE HEART DO?

The heart is an essential organ that pumps blood to the lungs to pick up oxygen and then pumps the oxygenated blood all around the body.

- It is a dual muscular pump. The right and left side of the heart are separated by the septum.
- It squeezes blood through one way valves in a network of narrowing arteries to the lungs and the rest of the body.
- The heart rate for an average male is between 60 to 80 beats per minute.
- It beats approximately 100,000 times/day (2,920,000,000 times in an average life span of eighty years).
- If it stops for just a few seconds, all hell breaks loose!

HEART ANATOMY

The heart has four chambers, the right and left atrium and the right and left ventricle (Figure 12.2).

The arteries carry blood *away* from the heart and the veins bring blood back to the heart. (Remember Artery begins with A for AWAY!). The arteries are therefore under greater pressure and have thicker walls. You will also feel a pulse in the arteries corresponding with the heartbeat but you will not be able to feel a pulse in a vein. This is because the pressure has dropped by the time the blood has travelled through the circulatory system from the heart via arteries to arterioles then to capillaries and then to venuoles before being transported back to the heart via the veins.

Blood that has been around the body and exhausted its supply of oxygen (deoxygenated blood) is transported back to the right side of the heart via the 85 *superior vena cava* (coming from the upper body) and the *inferior vena cava* (from the lower body).

It enters the right atrium and then travels through the tricuspid valve to the right ventricle. From here it leaves the heart via the right and left pulmonary arteries to the corresponding right or left lung.

In the lungs the pulmonary arteries become smaller arterioles and then even smaller capillaries. The capillaries have walls that are one cell thick and they form a mesh around the lower end of the airways where there are tiny dilated sacs called alveoli.

This is where inhaled oxygen can be transferred across the very thin walls of the airways and surrounding capillaries, into the blood stream. The alveoli are shaped like bunches of grapes to increase the surface area across which the gases can be exchanged and this makes the process more efficient (Figure 12.3).

Carbon dioxide (the waste gas produced from metabolism in all the organs of the body) is also transferred from the blood back into the airways to be exhaled.

The re-oxygenated blood is now transported back through the pulmonary veins to the left atrium. From here it travels through the mitral valve into the left ventricle. This is the largest chamber in the heart and when it contracts it squeezes the blood with its vital oxygen out through the aorta.

The aorta divides into an ascending aorta sending blood to the upper body, and the descending aorta, sending blood to the lower body.

This vital transport system can only be maintained if the heart beats at an appropriate rate.

WHAT MAKES THE HEART CONTRACT?

The heart is a muscle. Inside the right atrium there is an area of specialised heart tissue called the sinus node or sinoatrial (SA) node (Figure 12.1). This node produces an electrical impulse that travels down through the right atrium to another area of specialised tissue called the atrioventricular node. From here the electrical impulses travel down through the bundle of His and spread out around the heart muscle causing it to contract. When the ventricles contract the blood is pushed out through the arteries.

These electrical currents spread through the whole body. They can be picked up by applying electrodes to various parts of the body and connecting them to an electrocardiograph. So the ECG is a graphic recording of electrical processes that make the heart muscle contract.

Abnormalities result in changes in the ECG and can help with diagnosis depending on the extent and position of the changes.

> **The ECG detects the electrical current flowing through the heart and depending on the size and state of the heart muscle, it will produce deflections on the ECG monitor.**
>
> **It also shows the heart rate and rhythm.**

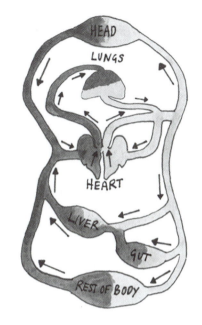

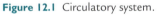
Blood carrying carbon dioxide in veins
Blood carrying oxygen in arteries

Figure 12.1 Circulatory system.

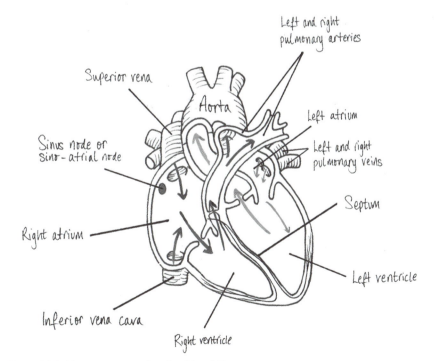

Left and right
pulmonary arteries

Superior vena

Aorta

Left atrium

Sinus node or
Sino-atrial node

Left and right
pulmonary veins

Septum

Right atrium

Left ventricle

Inferior vena cava

Right ventricle

Figure 12.2 Heart anatomy showing blood flow.

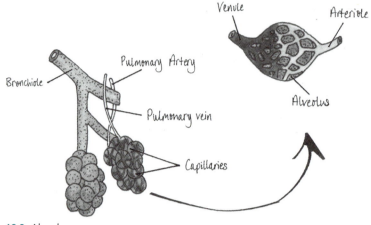

Venule

Arteriole

Pulmonary Artery

Bronchiole

Pulmonary vein

Alveolus

Capillaries

Figure 12.3 Alveolus.

PQRST

The electrical activity occurring in the heart is reproduced graphically on the ECG recording and is comprised of three waves that have been assigned the letters P, QRS, T (Figure 12.4).

- P represents the electrical activity during contraction of the smaller chambers (atria).
- QRS represents the current that causes contraction of the left and right ventricles. Because the ventricles have a larger muscle mass than the atria, there is a larger deflection on the ECG recording.
- T represents the repolarization (like resetting of the spring) of the ventricles. The repolarization of the atria is hidden in the QRS complex.

HEART DISEASE

Various types of heart disease that affect the heart muscle or interfere with the rate or rhythm may be detected on an ECG.

Remember the heart is a muscle so it also needs an independent blood supply to obtain its oxygen and nutrients. This is delivered via the right and left coronary arteries.

In heart disease these arteries may be narrow or blocked by fatty deposits called atheroma. This restricts the flow of blood to the heart muscle (*ischaemia*). The restriction is initially more of a problem when the heart muscle is working hard as in exercise or exertion. The heart needs more blood for its supply of oxygen and nutrients and if the blood supply is compromised the heart muscle will not be able to work properly and will become painful. This is what causes the pain of *angina* which is typically felt during exertion or stress. The pain will go after rest, unless there is a complete blockage or clot. In this case the pain will not go with rest as the affected muscle is completely deprived of oxygen (Figure 12.5) and it dies (heart attack or *myocardial infarct*).

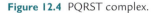

Figure 12.4 PQRST complex.

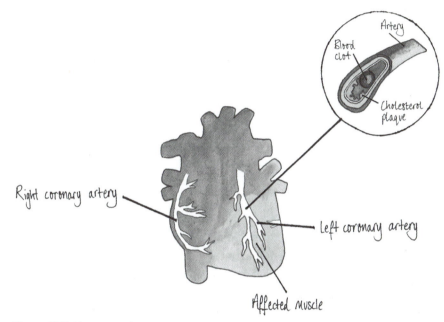

Figure 12.5 Heart attack.

When this happens the outcome will depend on where the blockage has occurred. If it is at the end of one of the tiny branches of the coronary artery it may only be experienced as a feeling of indigestion for a while (a silent heart attack), and this may only be detected on a subsequent ECG. If the blockage is further up the coronary artery it will affect a larger area of heart muscle and may cause the heart to stop (cardiac arrest) depending on the amount of heart muscle involved.

The pain of angina or a heart attack may be felt in the chest or jaw or left arm. Occasionally it may be felt in the right arm. This is because of the way in which the nerves are distributed in the chest wall. Other possible symptoms may include a feeling of pressure in the chest, indigestion, nausea, vomiting, sweating, shortness of breath, feeling dizzy or faint.

The ECG recording may look different in someone who has ischaemic heart disease or who has had a heart attack. This is because the muscle may be damaged so the flow of electric current through the muscle is altered and the deflections on the recording will be different.

ATRIAL FIBRILLATION (AF)

This occurs when the sinus node fires erratic impulses causing the atria to 'fibrillate' (beat very rapidly). This churns the blood up as it goes through the heart valves to the ventricles. It is a major cause of complications and death due to the formation of clots. It is also associated with valvular and ischaemic heart disease, hypertension, and heart failure, thyrotoxicosis, alcohol excess, and acute infections. Atrial fibrillation is associated with a number of complications such as difficulty breathing, blood clots, stroke, and congestive heart failure.

The ECG recording will look different in atrial fibrillation. Because the atria are not beating properly the P wave does not show up clearly on the ECG recording. It may only appear as a fibrillatory line like a series of small bumps. This is very characteristic of AF.

HEART FAILURE

This is when the heart cannot pump the full amount of blood with each heartbeat and is therefore unable to meet the needs of the body. It is classified as systolic and diastolic failure and may affect only the right ventricle or the left ventricle or both.

It is commonly caused by heart disease such as after a heart attack or may occur as a result of uncontrolled hypertension. It may also be a complication of atrial fibrillation or valve disease.

Around 900,000 people in the UK have heart failure. The incidence rises steeply with age and carries a poor prognosis that is actually worse than most cancers with 30–40% of patients diagnosed with heart failure dying within a year, usually because by the time it is diagnosed it is quite advanced (NICE 2010). It can only be definitely diagnosed by an echocardiogram and the Quality and Outcome Framework indicators encourage the echocardiogram as a target for all patients with suspected heart failure. This is to promote earlier diagnosis in an effort to treat the problem more quickly and prevent early complications.

There are many possible symptoms including shortness of breath, swelling of the feet and legs, a chronic lack of energy, difficulty sleeping caused by breathing problems, a swollen or tender abdomen and a loss of appetite, a cough with frothy sputum, increased urination at night and confusion or an impaired memory.

The ECG recording may show the possible *cause* of heart failure such as AF or a previous myocardial infarction and it may demonstrate possible signs of heart failure such as an enlarged left ventricle (left ventricular hypertrophy). It can be useful to signal the need for further investigations but it cannot provide a definitive diagnosis.

THE TWLEVE-LEAD ECG

When detecting any abnormalities in the current flowing through the heart, the ECG can determine *where* the abnormality may be. It does this by viewing the heart from different directions. To record an ECG there are six chest electrodes and four limb electrodes, but it becomes a little confusing as it is referred to as a twelve-lead ECG.

So how does 6 + 4 = a 12-lead ECG?

- A lead is a view of the electrical activity of the heart from a particular angle across the body, obtained by using signals from different combinations of electrodes.
- To obtain a twelve-lead ECG you have one electrode attached to each of the limbs, and six electrodes placed on the chest, ten in total but you get twelve "leads" or pictures from the combinations of different electrodes.
- For the chest, the six leads take their picture (or view) from an electrode each and are referred to as unipolar (Leads 1–6).
- Three of the limb leads are made up from the signals of two electrodes each and are referred to as bipolar (Leads l, ll, lll).
- The other three limb leads are made up from signals of three electrodes each and are called augmented leads (aVF, aVR, aVL).
- The electrode placed on the right foot serves only as an electrical earth and does not play a part in the recording.

Some reasons for performing an ECG:

The ECG can be useful monitoring patients with heart disease and to aid in diagnosis. It might be requested by the doctor for any one of the following reasons:

- Chest pain? Always make sure you have professional help at hand in case of sudden deterioration in the patient.
- History of chest pain or heart attack.
- Hypertension.
- Palpitations.
- Patient at risk.
- Prior to some drug treatments.
- Shortness of breath.

Recording an ECG: The process

(Adapted from the British Cardiovascular Society Guidelines 2010) Protocol! You can download the National Occupational Standard SFHCHS130 *Perform Routine Electrocardiograph Procedures* to use as a checklist for your competencies (Skills for Health 2011).

Preparing the patient (Figure 12.6):

Good preparation is an essential part of the process in the quest for the most accurate ECG recording.

1. Confirm the patient's identity, and make sure this correlates to the name on the computer screen.
2. Explain the process including what will happen before, during, and after the procedure. Ensure the patient understands and is happy to proceed (obtain informed consent).

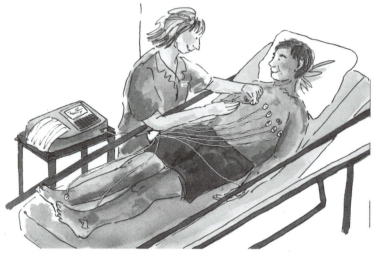

Figure 12.6 HCA performing ECG.

3. Consider privacy and comfort in what can be a distressing and embarrassing procedure for some patients. A chaperone should be offered according to the local policy.

4. The patient should be lying down with the head well supported. Patients who have breathing difficulties may need to sit in a more upright position and sometimes it will be necessary to perform an ECG on a patient in a wheelchair. Any variation from the supine position should be documented.

5. There should be unrestricted access to the chest, arms and legs. Remember to offer a "dignity blanket" for female patients to minimise embarrassment.

6. Reassure the anxious patient. Anxiety will make the heart beat faster so the result will not be accurate. Make sure they understand that the ECG is a recording of electrical activity from them and is not a current being passed through them!

7. If the skin is sweaty or oily, clean it with an alcohol wipe to ensure a good contact. Similarly if the patient has a lot of chest hair it is sometimes necessary to shave those areas where the electrodes are to be stuck on. Always use a disposable single use razor. If exfoliation is required, rub the skin lightly with an abrasive tape designed for the purpose.

8. Discourage any talking or movement as this involves the use of other muscles. Make sure the patient's fists are not clenched. All muscles contract because of electrical stimulus so there is the potential for this to interfere with the recording from the heart.

Positioning the electrodes:

9. It is important to place the electrodes consistently and in the best place to achieve the most accurate recording. Studies have shown that electrodes are frequently placed incorrectly producing significant diagnostic differences (Kligfield et al. 2007). Because of this there are recommended positions that should be adhered to if at all possible or if not then the alternative positions used should be documented. Electrodes on the limbs and chest should be placed as in **Box 12.1**. (See also Figure 12.7.)

Box 12.1. Recommended positions for the electrodes

Electrode	Recommended position
Red	Inside the right wrist
Yellow	Inside the left wrist
Green	Inside the left ankle
Black	Inside the right ankle
V1	4th right intercostal space at sternal border
V2	4th left intercostal space at sternal border
V3	Midway between V2 and V4
V4	5th left intercostal space in mid clavicular line
V5	Left anterior axillary line at same horizontal level as V4
V6	Left mid axillary line at same horizontal level as V4

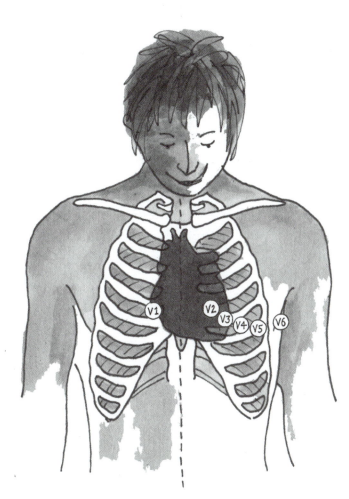

Figure 12.7 ECG leads on the chest.

Tips for remembering the limb leads:

It may be helpful to remember the sentence "Ride Your Green Bike" (RYGB) as a memory aid for the sequence of limb electrode colours. So the red electrode is applied to the inside of the right wrist, the yellow electrode is applied to the inside of the left wrist, green electrode to the left foot and black electrode to the right foot.

When a patient has a tremor or is an amputee it may be necessary to position the limb lead on the corresponding shoulder or lower torso. Always document any variation from the regular position.

Tips for placing the chest leads:

To identify the fourth intercostal space for the chest leads it may be helpful to slide a finger from the base of the throat downwards as far as a bony lump (Angle of Louis). Then slide the finger to the left or right to identify the appropriate fourth intercostal space. Alternatively count the dips in between the ribs starting at the clavicle and working downwards to the fourth dip.

Chest leads lll to V can be placed under or over breast tissue.

10. Once the electrodes have been applied and good contact ensured, press the button to start the machine and record a twelve-lead ECG at 25 mm/sec with a gain setting of 10 mm/mv. The filter setting should only be used if there is interference from other muscle movement and should be clearly marked on the recording. If the rhythm is irregular, an additional rhythm strip should be recorded usually on lead V2 for a minimum of 10 sec. This has to be done manually.
11. When the recording is done, ensure correct labelling and show it to the requesting practitioner before the patient leaves the surgery (or proceed according to the Local Protocol).
12. Scan it immediately onto the computer and make sure the paper recording is stored away from the clinical area to preserve confidentiality.

Other factors to consider

Infection control: Observe correct hand decontamination before and after the procedure, clean the couch between patients. Dispose of couch roll and disposable razors in line with your local policy.

Health and safety: Make sure the couch is at the correct height. Ideally couches in the treatment room should be adjustable so that the patient can get on and off safely and the practitioner can attend to the patient without bending. Take care when helping patients on or off the couch.

All electrical equipment should be checked annually and the date recorded on the equipment. It should also be calibrated annually or as recommended by the manufacturer.

Now try the quiz below – you can check back in the text if you've forgotten some of the answers.

HEART AND ECG QUIZ

1) List three reasons why a patient might need to have an ECG.
2) What are the fours chambers of the heart called?
3) Which blood vessels carry blood away from the heart?
4) Which vein carries blood back to the heart from the upper body?
5) Where do the pulmonary arteries carry the blood to and why?
6) Which area of the heart normally produces the electrical impulse that makes the heart muscle contract?
7) How should the patient be positioned to have an ECG?
8) Where would you place the electrode V2?
9) Where would you place the red electrode?
10) How do you get twelve leads (pictures) from ten electrodes?

Using a framework for reflection (see Chapter 2), try reflecting on a consultation where you performed an ECG recording. How did it go and what did you learn?

13

Venepuncture Best Practice

Venepuncture is a task that is often one of the first to be taken on by a HCA, and many will be extremely proficient in the procedure. It is, however, another one of those tasks where it is so essential to get it right in order to achieve the best and most accurate sample possible. This may sound obvious but it is surprising how many errors "competent" phlebotomists can make that can have significant implications for the patient. This chapter will provide some of the necessary underpinning knowledge in the physiological process and will outline the correct procedure to achieve accurate sampling.

Before you consider performing venepuncture, make sure you are up to date with your hepatitis B protection.

THE CLOTTING PROCESS IN VENEPUNCTURE

When a hole is made in the vein by the needle, platelets (small fragments of blood cells) become sticky and clump around the injury. Activated platelets and injured tissue produce chemicals that react with clotting factors in the blood. These clotting factors are known by the Roman numerals l to Xlll. Factor l (fibrinogen) is converted into thin strands of solid protein called fibrin. These strands trap the platelets and blood cells to form a solid clot or plug. This process may take several hours so it is important to remind the patient not to do anything after the procedure that may interfere with this or they risk further bleeding and subsequent bruising.

Factors that may interfere with the clotting process:

There are several factors that may affect the clotting of the blood.

- Abnormal liver function (the liver produces the clotting factors)
- Vitamin K levels (because Factors ll, Vll, IX and X are dependent on vitamin K)
- Clotting disorders such as haemophilia
- Anticoagulants such as aspirin, warfarin, heparin
- Hypercoaguability disorders
- Low-platelet counts such as in immunosuppression, leukaemia, platelet function disorders
- Heavy lifting or excessive movement within two hours of venepuncture

Order of draw

Blood samples should be drawn in the correct order to avoid cross contamination of additives between tubes (WHO 2010).

Check with your local laboratory for current guidelines regarding which colour sample bottles to use for which test and the order of draw. A general rule is that blood glucose samples should be taken last in the order of draw as these bottles contain an enzyme which may adversely affect other tests if there is any cross contamination.

FACTORS AFFECTING THE QUALITY OF THE SAMPLE

There are some factors that may affect the results of a blood sample that the blood taker cannot do anything about, such as the patient's age, gender, race, pregnancy and so on.

There are other factors that may affect the quality that will depend very much on the competence of the blood taker.

Haemolysis is the term used to describe the damage of red blood cells resulting in leakage of their contents into the blood plasma. Where a blood sample is haemolysed the test may give a falsely high reading for substances such as potassium. This is because most of the potassium in the body is intracellular (contained within the cells). When the cell is damaged the potassium leaks out into the serum, so the blood sample will give a false high reading. Potassium is very important for muscle contraction, particularly of the heart muscle, so patients who have a high potassium level will always need to be retested fairly promptly.

ACTIVITY

List as many things as you can you think of that may cause damage to the blood cells during and after venepuncture or that may give inaccurate results for other reasons.

How could this affect patient care? Check your answers at the end of the chapter (Box 13.1).

A BIT ABOUT TOURNIQUETS

Ideally you should use tourniquets with a quick and slow release mechanism. Position the tourniquet 10 centimetres (a hand width) above the intended puncture site. It should be loosened or removed when the first tube starts to fill and never left on for longer than is absolutely necessary.

Always remove the tourniquet before removing the needle from the vein.

If the vein is clearly visible and palpable, consider taking the blood *without* using a tourniquet. Prolonged use may be uncomfortable and can cause haemolysis, adversely affecting the quality of the sample.

Some research has identified contamination with MRSA on multiple use tourniquets (Elhassan and Dixon 2011). There is an ongoing debate about the need for disposable tourniquets. The problem with these is that they do not incorporate a slow release mechanism so they are either on or off. There is therefore no way to easily retighten the tourniquet if the blood flow stops.

If nondisposable tourniquets are used, then consider washing them at the end of every session, and never use them if they are visibly contaminated.

VENEPUNCTURE: THE PROCESS: PROTOCOL!

Choosing the best arm is seen in Figure 13.1. An example of venupuncture can be seen in Figure 13.2.

You can download the National Occupational Standard SFHCHS 132 *Obtain venous blood samples* to use as a checklist for your competencies (Skills for Health 2011).

1. Identify the patient by asking them to say their name and address and date of birth (you must have three points of reference)
2. Obtain informed verbal consent before proceeding
3. Check the history. Has the patient had any previous problems with the procedure or any surgery to one side where use of the opposite arm may be advised (e.g. lymph node clearance)? Have they fasted if necessary?
4. Position the patient appropriately. Always lie them down if they have fainted before or if they are unsure. The chair should ideally be designed for the purpose but failing this should, as a minimum requirement, have arms to prevent the patient falling to the side.
5. Decontaminate your hands and put on gloves
6. Prepare the equipment
   - Blood collection bottles according to the tests to be collected (charts with blood bottle colours are available from all hospital pathology laboratories). Always put a spare set of bottles on the tray in case there are problems obtaining the blood. Check that bottles are in date
   - Two needles (one spare): 20, 21 and 22 gauge needles are all suitable
   - Cotton wool ball
   - Alcohol wipe
   - Tourniquet
   - Plaster or hypoallergenic tape
   - Sharps box
   - Bottle holder (if using the vacuette system)
7. Identify the best arm and expose the antecubital fossa (inside the elbow)
   Avoid using the weak or paralysed arm if the patient has had a stroke. Any tight clothing should be removed. Support the patient's arm on a pad and advise the patient to keep the arm straight throughout the procedure. Look for the most visible and palpable or "bouncy" vein. The median cubital vein is usually the easiest to puncture. The basilic vein may be used but as it usually runs above the artery and nerve there is a greater risk of an arterial stab or nerve damage so it is best avoided if possible.

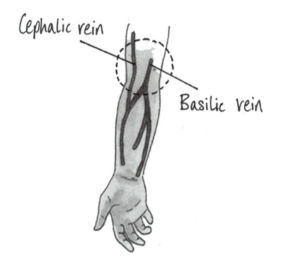

Cephalic vein

Basilic vein

Antecubital fossa

Figure 13.1 Antecubital fossa.

Where there isn't a good visible vein, apply the tourniquet and take time to carefully palpate the area to identify the best vein. Time taken at this stage is time well spent!

Try to avoid choosing a site where the veins are diverging as there is more risk of a bruise forming.

8. Now clean the area using an alcohol wipe working with a firm downward motion across the whole area for thirty seconds (WHO 2010).

9. While the alcohol dries, prepare the equipment.

10. Retighten the tourniquet *if necessary*.

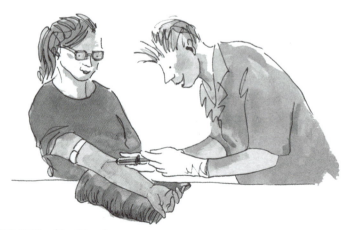

Figure 13.2 HCA taking blood.

Vacuette system (used in most areas in England and Wales):

- Attach the needle to the holder (vacuette).
- Drop the sheath off the needle at 90 degrees to avoid any spur on the needle that might occur if the sheath is pulled off horizontally.
- Warn the patient to expect a sharp scratch. Insert the needle, bevel upwards, into the vein at a 30-degree angle to about half the length of the needle.
- Push on the first bottle (observing the order of draw) while firmly anchoring the holder so that the needle doesn't move in the vein.
- When the blood starts to flow, loosen the tourniquet if it has been tightened. Allow the blood to finish filling the tube completely before gently removing and inverting the tube twice.
- Apply the next bottle and repeat the procedure.

Monovette system (used in some areas):

- Attach the needle to the first bottle (observing the order of draw) and twist to lock. Drop the sheath off the needle at ninety degrees to avoid any spur on the needle that might occur if the sheath is pulled off horizontally.
- Warn the patient to expect a sharp scratch.
- Insert the needle, bevel upwards, into the vein at a 30-degree angle to about half the length of the needle.
- Pull out the plunger of the bottle until it clicks, taking care not to move the needle in the vein.
- When the blood starts to flow loosen the tourniquet if it has been tightened.
- Allow the bottle to finish filling the tube completely before removing and inverting twice.
- Attach the next bottle and repeat. (Second and subsequent bottles can be prepared by pulling out the plunger until it clicks and then snapping it off).

Finishing up:

1. *Before* taking the needle out, remember to remove the tourniquet.
2. Remove the needle and then apply the cotton wool, advising the patient to press firmly for a few minutes (may need longer if on anticoagulant therapy).
3. Pick up all the bottles and invert fully again a further four times (so six in total).
4. Label the bottles checking details with the patient and put into the pathology bag/form.
5. Apply an appropriate dressing to the venepuncture site (always check for allergies first).
6. Dispose of sharps and equipment immediately, according to local policy.
7. Remove gloves and decontaminate hands.
8. Advise the patient about after-care and follow-up.
9. Document the procedure. Include consent obtained, which blood tests were taken, who the requesting practitioner was and any problems that were encountered.

TROUBLESHOOTING

What will you do if any of the following occur?

- **The patient faints during the procedure:** This depends on whether or not they are safe. If they are lying down and quite safe, continue with the procedure. It is much better to do this than to have to go through the whole procedure again if it makes them faint!

  If they are not safe, take off the tourniquet and remove the needle. Advise the patient to lean forward with their head down or to lie down. Apply a dressing to the venepuncture site. Support the patient gently to the floor if necessary and elevate the legs. Recovery from a simple faint is usually quite quick, but they may need a glass of water and observation for a short while. If the blood has not been taken at this stage, refer them to a registered practitioner for further tests. Always have the patient checked over by a registered practitioner before they leave the surgery if they have been unwell.

- **An artery is punctured instead of a vein:** This is an uncommon event but can happen especially when choosing a vein on the inner edge of the antecubital fossa. This is where the brachial artery is usually but it is deeper and can be distinguished from a vein because the artery will have a pulse and will not 'plump up' when the tourniquet is applied. Blood from an artery will pump into the collection bottle in spurts and will be a brighter red colour than that from a vein. If this happens, take the tourniquet off and remove the needle. *You* apply pressure for a minimum of five minutes and apply a pressure dressing when bleeding has stopped. Ask a registered practitioner to assess the patient before attempting venepuncture again or before the patient leaves the surgery.

- **The vein "collapses":** This usually means that the vacuum has sucked the wall of the vein onto the needle and stopped the flow of blood. This can sometimes be overcome by taking the bottle off and then reapplying or by gently tilting the needle in the vein.

- **There is no blood flow:** The needle may have gone through the vein or missed it completely. Gently and very slowly withdraw or manoeuvre the needle until the blood starts to flow. If there is still no success, slowly take the needle out checking all the time for any indication of blood flow. Repeat the procedure with a fresh needle and bottle. Do not make more than two attempts on each arm.

AN OVERVIEW OF SOME COMMON BLOOD TESTS

Full blood count (FBC): This tells us how many red blood cells, white blood cells and platelets there are. It also identifies the different types of white blood cells. The shape and size of the cells can be determined. *Red blood cells* carry essential oxygen attached to haemoglobin. Because of this, a reduction in the number of red blood cells or a problem with them can result in a shortage of oxygen in the body. *White blood cells* (made up of neutrophils, lymphocytes, monocytes, basophils, and eosinophils) fight different types of infection and are essential in the immune system. *Platelets* are small fragments of cells that are important in the clotting process.

The FBC is a haematological test and may be done for a number of reasons some of which are listed here:

- Hypertension (because too many red blood cells can make the blood thicker and increase the blood pressure)
- Heart disease
- COPD
- Diabetes
- Any prolonged or recurrent infection
- Cancer – undergoing chemotherapy
- Inflammatory diseases requiring disease modifying anti-rheumatic drugs (DMARDS) such as methotrexate
- Anaemia

Erythrocyte sedimentation rate (ESR)

Inflammatory processes affect the red blood cells and prolong the time it takes to spin them down in a centrifuge. So the ESR can indicate if there is any inflammation going on in the body. It will also be influenced by age and gender.

The ESR should be measured within two hours of the blood being taken to achieve the most accurate result.

Kidney or renal function test (RFTs), also referred to as urea and electrolytes (U&Es)

The kidneys are two small organs positioned either side of the back in the left and right loin. They are essential organs and act as filters for the blood, sieving out waste products and excreting them in the urine. When the kidneys are not functioning properly, toxic waste products can build up in the blood and interfere with the normal functioning of the body.

Kidney-function tests are performed to measure the levels of urea, creatinine and electrolytes including sodium, potassium, chloride, and bicarbonate. Some of the reasons for checking kidney function include:

- Kidney disease
- Hypertension
- Diabetes
- When the patient is taking specific medications such as some anti-hypertensives

The kidney function test will also identify the glomerular filtration rate (eGFR) which indicates the rate at which the kidney is filtering the blood and can therefore give information about the health and efficiency of the kidney.

Liver function tests (LFTs)

The liver is a vital organ in the right upper part of the abdomen. It has a number of essential functions:

- Storage of glycogen (made from sugars, this is the fuel for the body)
- Metabolising (break down) fats and proteins from food
- Processing and metabolising many toxins and drugs
- Production of vitamin K and other chemicals needed to help the blood clot
- Production of bile (stored in the gall bladder) which is necessary for digesting fats

LFTs measure the levels of liver enzymes, such as alkaline phosphatase (ALP), alanine transaminase (ALT), and aspartate aminotransferase (AST); abnormal levels may indicate liver disease. LFTs also measure albumin (the main protein produced by the liver), total protein, and bilirubin, which gives the bile its green-yellow colour and may make the patient look yellow (jaundiced) when there are high levels in the blood. Another test of the liver that may be done if requested is the gamma-glutamyl transferase (GGT or gamma GT). High levels may indicate alcohol abuse as well as other types of liver disease.

Some reasons for checking liver function tests are:

- To help diagnose and monitor liver disease
- As a precaution after starting some drugs such as statins, to check that they are not causing liver damage

Calcium

> Current literature advises against the use of the tourniquet when checking calcium levels as it has been suggested that prolonged use of the tourniquet gives a falsely high reading (Clinical Knowledge Summaries 2012).

Calcium is an essential mineral and about 99 percent is found in the bones and teeth with the rest found in the blood and soft tissues. It is vital for healthy bones and teeth and to help with muscle contractions, blood clotting, and nerve function.

Calcium levels may be checked in patients with:

- Kidney stones.
- Bone disease.
- Neurological (nerve) disease.
- Kidney disease.
- Symptoms of high calcium include fatigue, weakness, anorexia, vomiting, constipation, thirst, urinary frequency.
- Symptoms of low calcium include abdominal cramps, muscle cramps, tingling fingers.
- Other diseases that may be associated with abnormal calcium levels include thyroid disease, cancer, malnutrition, and intestinal disease.

Blood glucose

Diabetes is a disease where the body either does not produce any insulin or it may produce some, but the body is resistant to it. Insulin is a chemical that is produced by the pancreas and it is essential to enable glucose circulating in the blood, to enter the cells of the body in order for them to function properly. When the blood glucose cannot enter the cells, the levels in the blood will rise and subsequent high levels over time can cause many problems such as heart disease and strokes, eye damage, kidney damage, and numbness or pain in the feet and hands.

Diabetes is diagnosed by measuring blood glucose levels but in some areas it is now diagnosed by measuring the HbA1C.

A random blood glucose level of 11.1 mmol/L or more indicates diabetes. This will usually be confirmed with a fasting test.

A fasting blood glucose level of 7.0 mmol/L or more indicates diabetes but will usually be repeated to confirm the diagnosis.

When the levels are on the borderline and the diagnosis is in doubt, the patient will be referred for an oral glucose tolerance test. For this test the patient has to fast overnight and is then given a glucose drink. A blood sample taken two hours later showing a glucose level of 11.1 mmol/L indicates that the body is unable to deal efficiently with the glucose and confirms the diagnosis of diabetes.

HbA1C

When there is an excess of glucose in the system it will attach freely to haemoglobin in the red blood cells. Red blood cells live for about 120 days, so by measuring the haemoglobin that has glucose attached to it (glycated haemoglobin) this indicates the levels of circulating glucose in the blood stream over the past three to four months. It is much more useful to determine the overall diabetic control as a fasting glucose will only indicate the immediate glucose level.

Thyroid function tests

The thyroid gland is situated in the neck and it produces hormones that increase the body's metabolic rate and help to control the level of calcium in the blood.

Thyroid function tests are done to diagnose thyroid disorders and to monitor people who have an underactive thyroid gland (hypothyroidism) who take thyroid replacement medication (thyroxine). They are also done to monitor people who have an overactive thyroid (hyperthyroidism) and who take other types of drugs to counter the effects of this.

Newborn babies are checked for inherited thyroid problems.

The first test will usually be for the thyroid stimulating hormone (TSH) which is responsible for stimulating the gland to produce the hormones T4 and T3. Levels of these hormones will be checked if the TSH levels are abnormal.

Lipid profile test

Lipid is basically fat, and it is stored in the body as a source of energy. A lipid profile includes measurements of cholesterol, triglycerides, low density lipoprotein (LDL) and high density lipoprotein (HDL).

Cholesterol is a fat made in the liver from fats in the food we eat. We all need some cholesterol as it forms an important component of the cell walls in our body. It is carried in the blood stream by the lipoproteins HDL and LDL.

HDL is considered to be the transporter of "good cholesterol" as it may prevent the build-up of fatty deposits in the arteries (atheroma).

LDL is considered to be the transporter of "bad cholesterol" as it is the LDL that is mainly involved in the formation of atheroma.

Triglycerides are the end product of the metabolism of the bulky fats present in food. Triglycerides are stored in adipose (fat) cells to be used as energy if food is unavailable.

Hyperlipidaemia can occur in people who have an unhealthy diet but can also be inherited. It may be secondary to other conditions such as diabetes, thyroid disease and some liver and kidney disorders. It is an important risk factor for heart disease and strokes.

Diagnosis is usually made after a fasting blood test (fasting for twelve hours with only water to drink). High LDL levels are associated with a higher risk of heart disease and should be less than 3.0 mmol/L. However the ratio of total cholesterol to HDL (TC/HDL ratio) is also an important indicator and should be 4.5 or less.

International normalised ratio (INR)

This is a measure of how much longer it takes the blood to clot than normal so if the INR is measured as 2.0 the blood is taking twice as long as normal to clot. For most of us, assuming we are not taking any anticoagulant medication, our INR would be 1.0. The INR is a test used most commonly for patients who are taking warfarin.

Warfarin blocks the effects of vitamin K and depletes the clotting factors in the body so it inhibits the formation of clots which is useful in patient with some types of medical condition such as patients who have:

• Atrial fibrillation
• Deep vein thrombosis or pulmonary embolism
• Mechanical heart valves or heart valve disease

Each patient who takes warfarin will need an individualised specific dose which is titrated according to the INR result. An overdose of warfarin can have catastrophic effects resulting in the patient bleeding to death so the dose is absolutely critical and patients will require close monitoring.

Blood sample bottles for INR testing contain heparin which stops the blood from clotting so it can be tested accurately.

This principle applies to other blood tests as well – additives in the various blood sample tubes are measured for a specific amount of blood.

Always make sure that the blood sample bottle is filled to the mark on the tube. If the ratio of blood in the tube is too small for the amount of heparin additive in the tube, the INR will be recorded as much higher than it actually is. If you have difficulty 'bleeding' a patient, always document this on the form so that the laboratory staff can make allowances for this.

Now try the venepuncture quiz – you can check back in the text if you've forgotten some of the answers.

VENEPUNCTURE QUIZ

1) List two factors that might interfere with the clotting process.
2) Which blood bottle should be left until last in the "order of draw"?
3) What is haemolysis?
4) Assuming you have needed to use a tourniquet, when should you loosen it?
5) When should the tourniquet be removed completely?
6) What will you do if you puncture an artery in error?
7) How many points of reference do you need for labelling the bottles and form?
8) Why do we need red blood cells?
9) List two reasons why a patient may have a kidney function test
10) Why is it important to fill the blood bottle to the correct level?

CAPILLARY BLOOD TESTING

This is useful when only a very small amount of blood is needed or when venepuncture is difficult. It is a convenient way of monitoring blood glucose, INR and cholesterol levels.

It is not without potential pitfalls; however, and the person performing the test has to ensure that it is done correctly in order to provide as accurate a result as possible.

Capillary testing: The process protocol!

Using a framework for reflection (see Chapter 2), try reflecting on a consultation where you took blood from a patient. How did it go and what did you learn?

You can download the National Occupational Standard SFHCHS 131 *Obtain and test capillary blood samples* to use as a check list for your competencies (Skills for Health 2011):

1. Confirm the identity of the patient.
2. Obtain verbal informed consent.
3. Decontaminate your hands, put on your gloves and prepare the necessary equipment.
   - Glucose meter
   - Cotton wool or gauze
   - Appropriate test strip (check that they are in date)
   - Control solution
   - Appropriate device for puncturing the skin

- Clean tray to hold the equipment
- Sharps box

4. Make sure the patient's hands are clean, warm and dry before starting.
5. Remove strip from foil and insert into the meter with the three black lines at the end of the strip in the meter. The meter will turn on.
6. Check that the lot number matches the strip being used (if necessary).
7. Always use a fresh disposable lancet for each patient.
8. Select an appropriate area for puncture.
9. Use the middle, ring or little finger. Puncture the sides of the finger, parallel to the side edges of the nail. Try not to use the tip or pad of the finger because there are more nerve endings there and it will hurt more.
10. If performing the test for blood glucose, wipe away the first drop of blood and discard. Do not do this if checking the INR.
11. Squeeze gently until a rounded bead of blood is obtained. There must be sufficient blood for the meter to function accurately. Do not squeeze the finger too hard. The sample should flow freely from the puncture site. Compress the area then release for a few seconds and repeat. Take your time! If the flow is too slow you will need to apply a second puncture.
12. Touch the drop of blood to the white area at the end of the strip until the meter begins the test. Do not remove the test strip or disturb it during the count down.

Finishing up:

13. Once the sample has been obtained, ask the patient to apply pressure to the site with gauze and maintain pressure until the bleeding has stopped.
14. Dispose of all contaminated items in an approved container.
15. Remove your gloves and decontaminate your hands.
16. Document the result immediately and refer back to the doctor or nurse as necessary.
17. Ensure the meter is checked regularly with the local internal quality control tests and external quality control tests. (Contact your local laboratory for more information.)

Perform an internal quality control test:

- Daily on meters in use
- Weekly if meters not used often
- Whenever results seem odd
- To make sure the meter and strips are working properly
- Do not use the quality control solution if the expiry date has passed

Common sources of error:

Not puncturing the skin deeply enough
Not wiping away the first drop of blood (for testing glucose levels)
Squeezing too hard or milking the finger excessively
Using test strips that are past their expiry date
Using test strips that have been stored incorrectly and that are damp or damaged

Accuracy can also be affected by:

Poor peripheral circulation, i.e., poor blood flow to the fingers
Dehydration
Hypotension
Renal dialysis
Very high cholesterol levels greater than 13 mmol/L

Box 13.1. Poor practice in venepuncture.

Poor practice in venepuncture that may give inaccurate results:

- Using needles that are too small or too big

- Prolonged use of the tourniquet

- Delays in transit time after sampling

- Samples stored at wrong temperature, i.e., in an area that is too warm or too cold. Ideally samples should be stored in a cool box

- Using a thin or 'thready' vein

- Taking blood from a bruised area

- Not allowing antiseptic skin cleanser to dry

- Mixing samples incorrectly or not at all

- Bending needles

- Filling sample bottles from a syringe and needle

- Under-filling the sample

- Labeling the sample incorrectly

Patient care may be compromised as inaccurate or haemolysed results may result in inappropriate or delayed treatment. Repeat testing is uncomfortable and time consuming for patients and staff and is also costly.

14

Understanding Lung Function and Disease: Performing Accurate Lung Function Testing

Many HCAs are now being asked to perform lung function testing to assist the nurse in the chronic disease clinic managing patients with respiratory disease. This chapter will give an overview of the anatomy and physiology of the respiratory system and common respiratory diseases to enhance your understanding and enable you to perform lung function testing more efficiently and accurately.

WHY DO WE NEED TO BREATHE?

Breathing is something most of us take for granted and rarely think about unless we become short of breath for some reason.

Effective respiration provides us with essential oxygen which must then be transferred from our airways into the blood stream for distribution to all the organs and cells of the body. Oxygen is essential to help convert food into energy in our cells. This is called metabolism. Effective respiration also helps us to get rid of carbon dioxide which is a waste product of metabolism and which can become very toxic to the body if it accumulates.

When you inhale (breathe in), the diaphragm and muscles between the ribs (intercostal muscles), contract, and make the chest cavity expand. As the chest expands the pressure in the chest will drop and because the outside air pressure is now greater, air flows into the lungs. As you exhale (breathe out) the diaphragm and intercostal muscles relax, reducing the size of the chest cavity. This increases the pressure inside the chest so that air from inside the lungs, flows to the outside. The cycle is repeated every time you breathe.

Oxygen enriched air that we breathe in, travels down the trachea and is then sent via the left and right bronchus to the bronchioles in the lungs. The bronchioles become smaller and constantly branch so that if you looked at the inside of a healthy lung it would look something like the branches of a very dense tree in miniature. At the end of every tiny branch there is a tiny air sac called an alveolus (see Fig. 12.3). This is designed to maximise surface area for the exchange of gases (oxygen and carbon dioxide). From the outside it looks like a tiny bunch of grapes wrapped in capillaries which are tiny blood vessels. These contain de-oxygenated blood, in other words blood that has been all around the body and used up its oxygen supply. It is sent back from the heart to the lungs via the pulmonary artery, to collect more oxygen. The artery becomes smaller and smaller until it forms the mesh of tiny capillaries which are tiny blood vessels with very thin walls only one cell thick. The mesh of capillaries wraps intimately around the alveolus. Oxygen from the air in the alveoli can then diffuse across the cell walls and into the blood to be taken back to the left side of the heart and sent off around the body again. Carbon dioxide is transferred by the same mechanism in the opposite direction, back into the lungs and then exhaled.

Useful definitions

Tidal breathing: normal breathing where the volume of air entering and leaving the body of healthy adult will be about 500 ml.

Dead space: the inhaled air in the airways where no gaseous exchange can take place and it is usually about 150 ml.

Total lung capacity: the volume of air in the lungs following maximum inspiration, usually about 6 litres.

Residual volume: the air remaining in the lungs after full expiration.

LUNG DISEASE

Asthma

Asthma is a very common disease: 5.9 percent of the English population have asthma which is one of the highest rates in the world. Between 3 and 4.5 million people are affected with 1,000 to 1,200 deaths reported each year, 90 percent of which could probably have been prevented (DH 2011a).

So What Is It?

There is no standardised definition of the type, severity or frequency of symptoms, nor of the findings on investigation. There are various possible symptoms including wheeze, breathlessness, chest tightness, cough and of variable airflow obstruction. There may also be airway hyper-responsiveness and airway inflammation as components of the disease (British Thoracic Society [BTS] & Scottish Intercollegiate Guidelines Network SIGN 2012).

ACTIVITY

Please don't try this if you already have asthma - you already know what it feels like!

For those who have never had problems breathing, try taking in a little breath. Don't breathe out but take in another little breath and keep doing this until you can't breathe in any more. This is what it feels like not to be able to get any more air into your lungs.

It's quite frightening isn't it?

Asthma is very common, often misunderstood and often poorly managed. It can be very variable, very distressing and disabling, and can be life threatening, but most of the time it can be treated.

The airways may become twitchy and constrict easily. There might be swelling or inflammation or mucus in the airways as well which will make the airflow difficult. When the airways get smaller the person with asthma might cough or wheeze or have difficulty breathing. Sometimes they may feel as if their chest is tight or as if there is a band around the chest. This usually happens in response to a trigger and there are many possible triggers.

ACTIVITY How many possible triggers for asthma can you think of? Check your answers against those given in **Box 14.1.**

Asthma can occur at any age and tends to occur most often in people with other allergies or those who have a family history of asthma. Recent research indicates that if inherited it passes from mother to daughter and father to son (Hassan Arshad et al. 2012).

Treatment: Asthma can be treated with various inhalers and tablets and treatment follows a stepwise approach (BTS & SIGN Guidelines 2011), stepping up from occasional use of a bronchodilator inhaler (this will open up the airways), to regular use of inhaled steroids that help to stop the swelling and inflammation in the airways. Some patients will need very strong doses of inhaled steroids to control their symptoms and some may also have inhalers that give a long acting bronchodilator action. Whichever type of treatment they have, they should all be instructed by a nurse who has training in respiratory disease (or a doctor), on how to recognise their symptoms and manage them quickly and effectively. Never underestimate the potential danger in an asthma attack. All patients should seek emergency help if their symptoms are getting worse as asthma can become more severe very quickly.

Box 14.1. Triggers for asthma

Cigarette smoke (passive or active smoking)
Cold air
Pollen
Dust
Dust mite faeces
Animal hair
Chemicals such as solder fumes, glues, aerosols
Respiratory infection
Stress
Exercise
Laughter
Some medications such as beta blockers, nonsteroidal anti-inflammatories
Mould

CHRONIC OBSTRUCTIVE PULMONARY DISEASE (COPD)

Chronic obstructive pulmonary disease (COPD) is the fifth most common cause of death in England and Wales, accounting for more than 28,000 deaths in 2005 (NICE 2011b). The prevalence increases with age and is usually associated with smoking but can also have occupational causes such as exposure to dust or toxins. A small percentage of people with COPD may have inherited a condition called alpha 1 antitrypsin deficiency which results in destruction of the alveoli – the tiny air sacs at the end of the bronchioles.

In some disadvantaged sectors of community, e.g., people with schizophrenia, smoking prevalence is 74 percent and COPD presents a huge challenge (DH 2011a).

So what is it?

COPD is a term used to describe a number of conditions including chronic bronchitis, emphysema, chronic obstructive airways disease and chronic airflow limitation. Patients with COPD experience progressive breathlessness, chronic productive cough and limited exercise capacity. This is caused by airflow obstruction that is not reversible in the way that asthma is. There is permanent damage to the airways and treatment options are limited.

Managing COPD

Smoking cessation is the most important treatment, and it is never too late to stop despite what the patient may think. If the disease is in the early stages and symptoms are mild, no other treatment may be needed. Even if the patient has been a heavy smoker for most of their life, stopping smoking can still slow down the progression of the disease.

Treatments for Stable COPD:

Bronchodilator inhalers, e.g., salbutamol, terbutaline and salmeterol
Antimuscarinic inhalers, e.g., ipratropium and tiotropium
Steroid inhalers, e.g., beclometasone, fluticasone, budesonide
Combination inhalers
Bronchodilator tablets
Mucolytic medicines, which make the sputum less sticky and easier to cough up.

Treatments to manage exacerbations:

Steroid tablets to reduce the inflammation in the airways
Antibiotics
Admission to hospital

Treatments for end-stage COPD:

Domiciliary oxygen – this can only be prescribed by a hospital specialist.

Palliative care to keep the patient as comfortable as possible including physiotherapy and rehabilitation. Exercise training. Support and advice.

Medication for depression and anxiety may also be required.

The HCA role in caring for patient with COPD is an important one and includes:

- Promoting healthy living
- Monitoring bloods, blood pressure, lung function testing, pulse oximetry
- Encouraging influenza and pneumococcal vaccination
- Supporting patients and carers
- Referring patients with early signs or increasing problems
- Recognising and referring patients with associated depression and anxiety
- Keeping up to date with current developments and guidelines

LUNG FUNCTION TESTING

Peak flow recording

The peak flow measures the fastest rate of air blown out of the lungs in litres per minute. It can be used in the diagnosis and monitoring of asthma. Readings are dependent on the height, age and gender of the patient and a normal range can vary by up to 100 litres per minute more or less than the predicted level. A chart with normal peak flow values is available at: http://www.peakflow.com/top_nav/normal_values/

Recording the peak flow: The process!

You can download the National Occupational Standard SFHCHS19 *Undertake Routine Clinical Measurements* to use as a checklist for your competencies (Skills for Health 2011):

1. Check the patient's identity and obtain informed consent.
2. Decontaminate your hands.
3. Ideally the patient should be standing or sitting upright so that the lungs can fully expand.
4. Insert a disposable mouthpiece with a "one-way" valve into the peak flow meter. Use the appropriate size mouthpiece according to the age of the patient.
5. Set the pointer on the meter to zero and ask the patient to hold the meter underneath so their hands do not interfere with movement of the pointer.
6. The patient should then take a full breath in, seal their mouth around the mouthpiece, and blow hard and fast over one to two seconds.
7. Try to ensure that the patient remains upright when blowing. The natural tendency is to lean forward when blowing, but this will interfere with the lung expansion and deflation and the reading will not be accurate.
8. Always repeat the process three times and record the best of the readings. It is often useful to demonstrate the procedure to the patient using your own mouthpiece.

9. Sometimes patients cannot perform this procedure properly and if this is the case you must document it. If in doubt seek advice from the nurse.
10. Document the measurement, and report any low readings.

Spirometry

Asthma and COPD can be diagnosed by performing spirometry to measure how quickly and effectively the lungs can be emptied and filled. Measurements include:

- The amount of air the patient can blow out quickly and forcibly, i.e., the forced expiratory volume in one second = FEV1.
- The total amount blown out in one breath, i.e., forced vital capacity = FVC.
- FEV1/FVC. A low value indicates narrowed airways.
- The degree of reversibility following administration of a bronchodilator, e.g., salbutamol/age, height and gender will affect lung volumes.

COPD is categorised as mild, moderate or severe depending on the result.

- Mild (stage 1) FEV1 is at least 80 percent of the predicted value.
- Moderate (stage 2) FEV1 is 50 to 79 percent of the predicted value.
- Severe (stage 3). FEV1 is between 30 to 49 percent of the predicted value.
- Very severe (stage 4) FEV1 is less than 30 percent of the predicted value.

Performing Spirometry: The Process: Protocol!

Prior to the procedure the patient should have been advised not to smoke for at least an hour before – preferably twenty-four hours if possible, not to have had a heavy meal for at least two hours, not to have had an alcoholic drink for at least four hours, not to have had any vigorous activity for thirty minutes, and not to wear restrictive clothing. Any deviations from these requirements should be documented.

If the patient is attending for routine monitoring they can have their inhalers as usual. If they are attending for reversibility testing, they should have no short acting bronchodilator for four hours, no long acting bronchodilator for twelve hours, and no sustained release bronchodilators for twenty-four hours (Figure 14.1).

1. Check the patient's identity and obtain informed consent.
2. Decontaminate your hands before and after the procedure.
3. Check that there are no contraindications (Box 14.2).
4. Make sure they have an empty bladder!
5. Record age, gender, and height.
6. Patient should be seated in a chair with arms. Both their feet should be flat on the floor.
7. Advise the patient to loosen any tight clothing and remove any false teeth if they are loose fitting.
8. Perform the slow vital capacity before the forced vital capacity. This is done first because the airways will be likely to collapse prematurely when the patient with COPD tries to blow out hard. Place a nose clip on the patient or ask them to hold their nose. Ask the patient to breathe in as deeply as they can, place

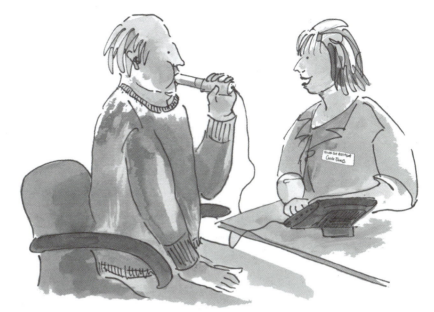

Figure 14.1 HCA performing spirometry.

Box 14.2. Contraindications to spirometry (*procedure should not be performed*)

Previous problems when performing spirometry

Current active chest infection

Current acute illness which could interfere with the ability to perform the test properly

Patient has been coughing up blood

Suspected or active TB

Unstable heart disease/angina

Recent pneumothorax (3 months)

Recent eye surgery

Recent abdominal or chest surgery (3 months)

Diagnosed aneurysm (thoracic, abdominal, or cerebral)

Refer back to the registered nurse if the patient has ear problems, has a history of fainting, has a diagnosis of glaucoma, or is pregnant

their lips around the mouthpiece to form a seal and then to blow out slowly and steadily for as long as they can. This is almost like sighing. Repeat this twice if possible to ensure the results are consistent, accurate and reproducible.

9. **Now perform the forced vital capacity.** Remove the nose clip. Ask the patient to blow out forcibly and rapidly for as long as they can until they have no breath left to blow out. This should take between six to fifteen seconds. Take a minimum of three readings if possible. The best two readings should have the FVC within 100 mls of each other.

10. The patient may need encouragement to keep blowing until they cannot blow anymore and it is helpful to place a hand lightly on their shoulder to stop them from leaning forward. This is a normal response in an effort to get every last breath out, but by doing this they will inadvertently compress the lungs a little and render the result inaccurate.

11. Advise the patient not to cough or take another breath during the procedure as this will invalidate the result. You can usually tell when this has happened as there will be a characteristic step in the flow graph. These results should be discarded and the test done again.

12. Stop the procedure and seek advice if the patient feels unwell at all during the procedure and seek advice from the nurse or doctor.

13. Some machines may require daily calibration in which case you should ensure that the date of calibration matches the date of the test. Follow the manufacturer's guidelines for calibration.

14. Record:
   • FEV1 and the percentage of the predicted FEV1
   • FVC and percentage of predicted FVC
   • Peak Flow (PEF)
   • FEV1/FVC

Reversibility Testing:

This only needs to be done if there is doubt over the diagnosis and to identify asthma.

1. The patient should be prescribed a bronchodilator inhaler (usually salbutamol).
2. Measure the FEV1.
3. The patient should then take four puffs of the inhaler via a large volume spacer.
4. After twenty minutes, remeasure the FEV1. If there is an increase of >12 percent from the baseline reading, this indicates reversible airflow obstruction and supports the diagnosis of asthma.

HCAs and nurses should not administer salbutamol unless it has been prescribed for the individual patient.

Now try the quiz below. You can check back in the chapter for the answers.

LUNG FUNCTION QUIZ

1) Why do we need oxygen?
2) What is the purpose of the alveolus?
3) What is meant by total lung capacity?
4) List three possible symptoms of asthma
5) How many readings should you take when performing a peak flow rate?
6) What is the most common cause of COPD?

7) What does FEV1 stand for?

8) What does a low value of FEV1/FVC indicate?

9) Why should you perform a slow vital capacity before the forced vital capacity?

10) Which inhaler will be prescribed for the patient to perform reversibility testing?

 Using a framework for reflection (see Chapter 2), try reflecting on a consultation where you performed lung function testing. How did it go and what did you learn?

Kidney Function and Urine: Performing Accurate Urinalysis

15

Why write a chapter on urinalysis? Surely it just involves dipping a test strip into a pot of urine and reading the result? What could be difficult about that? Of course there is much more to it, and in reality it is an important diagnostic tool that is all too often very badly performed resulting in inadequate or inaccurate information and a potentially incorrect diagnosis. As with any other task the HCA performs it is always easier to perform it well and accurately if there is an understanding of what is being tested for and why.

Urine has historically been used for many different things, and it has had many magical qualities attributed to it. Some tribes in Siberia drink the urine of people who have eaten magic mushrooms in the belief that this will help them communicate with the spirits. Ancient Romans used urine to bleach clothes. It has been used as an antiseptic and as a teeth whitener and is thought by many different cultures to cure any number of ailments such as acne, warts, hair loss, wrinkles, and gastric upset to name but a few!

Most importantly though, is the fact that urine testing can tell us a great deal about a person's general health.

What do the kidneys do?

We have two kidneys both weighing about 160 g and measuring 10 to 15 cm long. They filter the toxins and waste products from the blood and these are then excreted in the urine.

Each kidney contains approximately two million microscopic sieves or filtering systems called nephrons which consist of networks of capillaries called glomeruli where the first phase of filtration occurs. The Bowman's capsule surrounds each glomerulus and is connected to a long tube or "tubule." The kidney receives about one litre of blood every minute. This blood is filtered through the nephrons and the resulting fluid is sent through the long tubule where most of the water, essential salts such as potassium, sodium and other substances such as glucose, amino acids and vitamins are reabsorbed back into the bloodstream. The remaining water, urea and other waste substances make up the urine and this is passed down the ureter to the bladder. Urine is normally made up of 5 percent salts and ammonia and 95 percent water.

Approximately two litres of urine are produced in twenty-four hours but this can vary greatly and depends on factors such as fluid intake, sweating, and general health.

The kidneys are essential for maintaining homeostasis – the normal balance of fluids and salts or electrolytes upon which the proper functioning of the body depends.

The kidneys also secrete some essential hormones such as erythropoietin that is needed to make red blood cells. So patients with kidney failure may become anaemic (lacking in oxygen) if they fail to produce enough of this hormone and therefore lack red blood cells to carry the oxygen.

The nephrons are very delicate structures and easily damaged especially when pressures are increased such as in hypertension or where the renal artery supplying the kidney with blood is narrowed (renal artery stenosis). When they are damaged, the sieves or filters become leaky and larger molecules such as proteins (not normally seen in urine) may become detectable.

What can urine testing tell us?
Look at it

Normal urine is straw coloured and transparent. So first of all have a good look at it and assess if the sample looks normal.

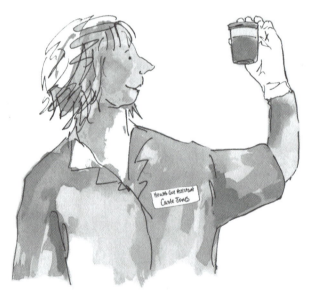

Is it dark or pale? If it is very pale it indicates a good level of hydration. If very dark it may indicate dehydration.

What colour is it? The colour of the urine can also be altered by medication, foodstuff and disease. Red or pink urine may indicate blood but may also be caused by eating beetroot! Bright yellow urine can be caused by some vitamins and other medications. Brown urine may indicate the presence of bilirubin if, for example, there is gall bladder disease, but it may also be caused by iron supplements. Turbid or cloudy urine may indicate infection. Frothy urine can be due to the presence of glucose or protein.

So before you have even opened the urine bottle you may already have some idea of the health, hydration (or diet!) of the patient.

Smell it

Once you've opened the urine bottle, notice if there is any offensive smell.

A faecal smell could mean that there is a fistula or direct connection between the bowel and bladder where faeces is able to contaminate the urine. A fruity, sweet smell could be significant in a diabetic patient who may have ketoacidosis. If the urine smells of asparagus it is probably because the patient has been eating asparagus! An unpleasant strong smell of ammonia could be due to a bacterial infection.

Dip it

The presence of various substances in the urine that can be detected on the diptest can be very useful to the clinician in making a diagnosis.

Protein should not normally be present in any significant amount and anything greater than a trace could be significant so you must take care to observe the colour on the diptest carefully and record the result as accurately as you can. An early morning sample is the best when testing for protein.

Protein may be present in:

- Hypertension
- Kidney disease
- Infection
- Inflammation and malignancy
- Diabetes
- Pregnancy – indicating possible pre-eclampsia which is a medical emergency
- Pyrexia
- Dehydration
- After vigorous exercise
- "Orthostatic proteinuria" which is usually harmless and can sometimes be seen in children later in the day

Blood is not normally present. Take care when reading the test strip that you allow long enough for the reaction on the strip to occur. For blood this can take up to two minutes.

Blood may be present in:

- Infection
- Trauma or injury to the urinary tract or kidneys
- Kidney stones
- Malignancy

It may also be present:

- If the patient is menstruating
- After vigorous exercise

- After smoking or toxic chemical exposure
- With no known cause – but it should always be reported and investigated.

Ketones are produced by the breakdown of fatty acids.

Ketones may be present in:

- Uncontrolled diabetes – so the nurse or doctor should always be informed
- Anorexia or starvation
- Diarrhoea and vomiting
- Pregnancy
- Eclampsia
- Alcoholism

Nitrites can be caused by the reaction of some bacteria on urinary nitrates. The pink colour must be uniform to indicate a positive result.

Nitrites may be present when there is:

- Infection. However the test is highly sensitive to air exposure and will commonly give a false positive result so some laboratories no longer consider it relevant when deciding if further culture and sensitivity testing is required.

Leucocytes are white blood cells that are usually produced in response to infection.

Leucocytes may be present when there is:

- Infection or inflammation in the genito-urinary tract. There may be false positive results if the test is contaminated by vaginal discharge.

Specific gravity (SG) is often overlooked as a useful test but can demonstrate the concentration of solutes in the urine.

A low SG might indicate:

- Excessive fluid intake
- Renal failure
- Pyelonephritis
- Diabetes insipidus (this is a condition where there is a problem with the adrenal glands resulting in an inability to control the fluid balance. It is not to be confused with diabetes mellitus)

A high SG shows that the urine is very concentrated with a high level of solutes and could occur in:

- Dehydration
- Renal artery stenosis
- Heart failure
- Liver failure

The pH of the urine stands for the "potential of hydrogen" and demonstrates the concentration of hydrogen ions. This determines whether the urine is alkaline or acidic. Tap water and normal urine will usually be neutral with a pH of approximately 7.

A pH lower than 7 (acidic urine) may be found:

- In acute starvation
- In diabetic ketoacidosis
- When potassium levels are low
- When the diet is very acidic

A pH higher than 7 (alkaline urine) may be found:

- When potassium levels are high
- In a vegetarian diet

Bilirubin is a by-product of the breakdown of red blood cells and it is normally excreted in the bile. **It may be present in urine:**

- In liver disease or obstruction of the gall bladder

URINALYSIS: THE PROCESS: PROTOCOL!

You can download the National Occupational Standard SFHCHS7, *Obtain and test specimens from individuals* to use as a checklist for your competencies (Skills for Health 2011).

1. Always wear gloves.
2. Consider eye protection.
3. Check the expiry date on strips.
4. Immerse the test strip completely in the urine.
5. After dipping in urine, remove any excess urine by tapping the test strip gently on the top of the bottle.
6. Lay the test strip flat on a dry surface.
7. Always check the time and be patient. Some reactions can take up to two minutes. If you do not observe this simple rule you may miss potentially important results.
8. Do not discard urine until sure it will not be needed again.
9. Follow infection control procedures and wash hands thoroughly after removing gloves.
10. Document results accurately.
11. Inform requesting clinician as necessary.

Now try the quiz below and see how you get on. You can check back in the chapter if you have forgotten the answers.

URINALYSIS QUIZ

1) What do the kidneys do?
2) What factors might influence the amount of urine produced?
3) What does homeostasis mean?

4) What could cloudy urine indicate?

5) List two conditions that may cause proteinuria (protein in urine).

6) List two conditions that may cause haematuria (blood in urine).

7) Why should you report ketones in the urine?

8) How long should you wait before reading the test strip?

Using a framework for reflection (see Chapter 2), try reflecting on an episode when you performed a urine dip test. How did it go and what did you learn?

16

Skin and the Healing Process: Basic Wound Care

Before you can embark on basic wound care, you need to have an understanding of the skin and how it heals. Skin is the largest organ in the body – about two square metres in volume, weighing about six pounds. It basically keeps the outside out and the inside in! There are three layers in skin and each has specific functions.

SKIN ANATOMY

Epidermis: this is the outermost layer that protects the body from the elements. It prevents the entry of harmful microorganisms and can dispose of harmful pathogens. It prevents loss of fluid and also contains melanin cells. These cells give the skin its colour and protect the body from ultraviolet light.

Dermis: this is the layer of skin under the epidermis containing the nerve endings, blood vessels, oil glands, sweat glands as well as collagen and elastin which give skin its strength and elasticity, sadly lacking as we get older. The dermis regulates the body temperature through sweating and vasodilation (opening up) and constriction (closing down) of the capillaries near the surface. Pre-vitamin D3 is formed in the dermis during exposure to sunlight and this is then rearranged to form vitamin D3. This is necessary to regulate the concentration of calcium and phosphate in the bloodstream, promoting healthy bones.

Subcutaneous fat: this is the loose connective tissue largely made up of fat cells called adipocytes. It stores energy as lipids, helps keep the body warm, acts as a shock absorber, holds the skin to the underlying tissues, and houses the hair follicles.

THE PHYSIOLOGY OF WOUND HEALING

It is worth stopping to think sometimes about everything that is going on in your body without you even realising. When you cut a finger or if you sustain a much larger wound, the body sets to work immediately to clean and heal the wound. It is quite amazing how efficient the body can be at looking after us even when we may not be very good at it ourselves!

Haemostasis (meaning the stopping of blood flow) is the body's natural response to injury. The damaged blood vessels temporarily constrict thus stopping the bleeding. Activation of the clotting mechanism occurs resulting in the release of chemicals called clotting factors which are identified by the Roman numerals l to Xlll. Factor 1 called fibrinogen is converted to solid strands of protein called fibrin. The platelets become sticky and clump around the injured tissue. These are then reinforced by the strands of fibrin forming platelet plugs, sealing the injury and initiating healing.

Stage 1: The inflammatory phase

This lasts between 0 to 5 days and begins the healing response. There may be heat, redness, swelling and pain at this stage. White blood cells collect in large numbers at the site of injury and proceed to remove dead tissue, foreign material and pathogens from the wound. Pathogens can be bacteria, viruses or fungal organisms that are present in sufficient quantity and in the right environment to be able to cause infection. In wounds the pathogens are usually bacteria and only rarely include fungi or viruses (Collier 2004).

At this stage, yellow slough may appear on the wound surface and there may be redness around the wound. This is normal *at this stage* and should not be confused with infection.

Stage 2: Proliferation/Granulation phase

This usually goes on between days 3 to 14 and may overlap with the first phase. This is an important phase in wounds where there is skin loss. Tiny new blood vessels (capillaries) form in the dermis to supply blood with essential nutrients and oxygen and the wound bed granulation can then begin. The healing "granulating" tissue should appear to be bright red 'beefy' and moist. As long as the wound bed is moist, new pale pink skin cells (epithelial cells) can multiply and migrate across the wound bed in a process called *epithelialisation*. This process is delicate and easily hindered if the wound bed is not moist or if it is exposed to any further trauma during wound cleansing or during the removal of old dressings.

Stage 3: Maturation phase

This can begin at day 7 and last up to 12 months. There is a progressive reduction in the blood supply to the scar. Collagen fibres become bigger and reoriented to improve the strength of the new skin. The scar becomes paler and should eventually flatten and soften.

TYPES OF HEALING

The healing process is classified according to the type of wound.
• **Primary healing:** Also called *first intention healing*, this occurs when the wound closes by the coming together of the wound edges either spontaneously or with intervention such as with sutures or clips.

- **Secondary healing:** This occurs where there has been tissue loss. The wound heals by the process of epithelialisation (see under Stage 2 above) and wound contraction. There is no surgical intervention.

FACTORS AFFECTING HEALING

ACTIVITY

There are many different factors that can affect the healing process.
List as many things as you can you think of that may delay healing.
How could this affect patient care?

Check your answers at the end of the chapter (Box 16.1).

Problems in the Healing Process

An essential part of basic wound care is the ability to recognise what is normal and when there may be problems.

Clinical Signs of Infection

All wounds will have microorganisms present but this does not necessarily mean that the wound is infected. Routine wound swabbing may therefore provide erroneous and misleading results.

The microbial numbers in a wound can range from contamination to colonisation, terms which describe the normal situation where there is no associated ill health, through to critical colonisation and ultimately infection which are abnormal states resulting in an adverse host reaction (Kelly 2003). Wound swabbing should only be carried out when there are clinical signs of infection.

There are some important signs to look out for that may indicate problems in the healing process or possible infection and these should always be reported to the registered nurse or doctor immediately.

Signs indicating possible infection:

- Wound increasing or not reducing in size
- Increasing pain
- Heat
- Erythema (redness)
- Cellulitis
- Oedema (swelling)
- Wound breakdown
- Malodour (bad smell)
- Increased exudate (fluid leaking from the wound)
- Fragile granulation tissue – wound bleeds easily
- Systemic signs of fever and malaise, pyrexia.

TAKING A WOUND SWAB: THE PROCESS PROTOCOL!

The decision on whether to perform a swab should be made by the registered nurse or doctor but the task may be performed by the HCA. Follow these simple steps to ensure accurate sampling

1. Explain the procedure to the patient and obtain informed consent.
2. Decontaminate hands and put on gloves.
3. Irrigate the wound if necessary to remove slough, necrotic tissue or dried exudate. Irrigate using tap water or sterile saline. The wound may also be moistened if it appears dry as this will improve the 'catch' of the swab. There is little to be gained from swabbing a dry wound. Alternatively the swab tip can be moistened with sterile saline prior to performing the swab. Sterile cotton or rayon tipped swabs in a charcoal medium are recommended (Human and Jones 2004).
4. Move the swab across the wound bed in a zig-zag motion at the same time as rotating the swab between the fingers, covering as large an area of the wound as possible, working away from the area that is cleanest. Include material from the wound bed and wound margin (Cooper 2010).
5. Immediately place the swab back into the container with the transport medium.
6. Remove your gloves and decontaminate your hands.
7. Label the sample correctly and complete the necessary documentation to send with it. Include any relevant comments about the patient's general condition, type of wound etc.
8. Record in the patient notes.
9. Ensure transport of the swab to the laboratory as soon as possible (ideally within four hours).

Choosing the wound dressing

Each patient should have a clear care plan drawn up by the registered nurse at the initial assessment of the patient and their wound. The care plan will specify the type of dressing to be used and the frequency of dressing change. Most patients should be reviewed by the registered nurse regularly throughout the course of their treatment but the frequency will depend on the severity of the wound. Always refer back to the nurse if there are any problems or changes in the patient's condition.

Before deciding on the wound dressing the nurse should consider:

- The patient, their health status, environment, and mobility
- The wound type, size, and cause
- Allergies or intolerance
- Dressing efficacy (based on evidence)
- Cost
- Acceptability to patient and prescriber
- Local wound care formulary

ACTIVITY

Considering what you now know about the skin and the healing process, can you list the qualities of the ideal wound dressing?

Check your answers at the end of the chapter (Box 16.2).

There are many different wound **dressings** and intelligent use of the appropriate dressing can speed up the healing process. The choice of dressing should always be guided by the local wound care formulary as this will have been based on current available, unbiased and robust evidence.

ACTIVITY

Look up your local wound care formulary or contact your local tissue viability nurse, who will tell you where you can obtain a copy. You must be able to justify the use of dressings that are not included in the local formulary. Table 16.1 gives a list of dressings as listed in some wound care formularies and outlines their qualities and suitability for various wounds.

Remember dressings should be prescribed for individual patients and are for single use only. They should not be resealed and used again.

WOUND DRESSING: THE PROCESS: PROTOCOL!

You can download the National Occupational Standard SFHCHS12, *Undertake treatments and dressing related to the care of lesions and wounds* to use as a checklist for your competencies (Skills for Health 2011).

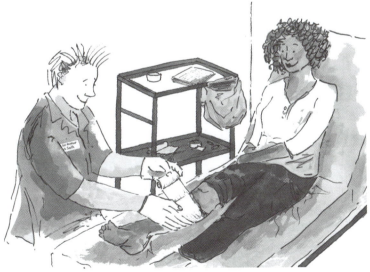

Figure 16.1 HCA performing wound dressing.

Remember:

• Always use a clean trolley.
  Wash hands before, after, and at any point during the procedure if hands become contaminated.

Table 16.1 Types of dressing: *follow the manufacturer's guidelines to apply the dressing correctly.*

Category	Qualities	Suitable for:	Points to consider	Example
Simple contact	Nonabsorbent, low adherence. Sometimes require a secondary dressing.	Low-exuding wounds. Fragile, delicate skin. Skin tears in the elderly.	Not suitable for heavily exuding wounds.	Atrauman Urgotul Mepitel
Semi-permeable film membranes	Permeable to water vapour and oxygen but impermeable to liquid. Transparent.	Wounds with little or no exudate, e.g., minor operation wounds healing by primary intention.	Not suitable for heavily exuding wounds.	C-view
Hydrocolloids	Absorb water to form a gel – maintain a moist environment. Can facilitate rehydration and debridement of dry sloughy or necrotic wounds.	Granulating or necrotic wounds, low to moderate exudate.	Avoid in diabetic foot wounds, caution in infected wounds as hydrocolloids can encourage the growth of anaerobic bacteria.	Hydrocoll Comfeel Plus Duoderm
Alginates	Will change to a gel in the presence of exudate. Highly absorbent. Haemostatic (stop bleeding). Debriding action. Require a secondary dressing.	Lightly exuding or bleeding wounds. Acute surgical wounds. Cavity wounds.	Not suitable for dry or necrotic wounds. Should not be used with antimicrobial or antibiotic creams or ointments as these may prevent the gelling process. Should never be left in a wound – all traces should be removed. Can cause maceration and excoriation of surrounding skin.	Kaltostat Sorbsan

(Continued)

Table 16.1 (Continued) Types of dressing: *follow the manufacturer's guidelines to apply the dressing correctly.*

Category	Qualities	Suitable for:	Points to consider	Example
Hydrofibre	Absorbs and interacts with wound exudate to form a soft hydrophilic gas permeable gel. Traps bacteria. Requires a secondary dressing.	Exuding lesions.	Very lightly exuding wounds may need to be moistened with sterile water or saline before application of the dressing. Not suitable for dry, necrotic wounds.	Aquacel
Silver dressings	Anti microbial action.	Should only ever be considered for critically colonised and infected wounds (Drugs and Therapeutics Bulletin 2010).	If no improvement is noted within 2 weeks replace with non-silver product.	Acticoat 3 or 7
Foams	Good absorption. Provide mechanical protection. May be used as a secondary dressing.	Exuding wounds (vary in absorption according to product used). May be beneficial in hypergranulating tissue.	Not for dry wounds. Always select appropriate size.	Activheal non adhesive foam 3M tegaderm foam Biatain Urgocell TLC
Odour absorbent dressings	Absorb odour.	Malignant fungating wounds and where there is anaerobic infection with an unpleasant odour.	Avoid unnecessary use.	Clinisorb Carboflex
Paraffin gauze	Reduces adherence of the dressing to the granulating wound. Requires secondary dressing.	Burns, ulcers, traumatic injuries, skin grafts.	Beware of maceration to surrounding skin in a heavily exuding wound. May become adherent if left on for too long.	Jelonet

(*Continued*)

Table 16.1 (Continued) Types of dressing: *follow the manufacturer's guidelines to apply the dressing correctly.*

Category	Qualities	Suitable for:	Points to consider	Example
Cadoxemer iodine	Absorbs exudate. Debriding action. Reduces microbial load. Requires secondary dressing.	Lightly exuding wounds at risk of infection.	Avoid in pregnant patients or those with thyroid disorders, or on lithium therapy. Take care in patients with iodine sensitivity. May cause stinging or burning. Treatment should not exceed 3months. Swabs should not be taken from wounds that have been dressed with iodine.	Inadine Iodofelx
Honey	Antibacterial action. Debriding and anti-inflammatory properties. Maintains moist wound bed. Reduces odour. Stimulates growth of new capillaries and skin cells. May require secondary dressing.	Open wounds healing by secondary intention. May increase exudate.	May cause stinging, burning.	Algivan Mesitran Medihoney
Zinc paste bandages	Cooling and soothing. Provide a moist wound environment.	Varicose eczema.	Must be applied correctly, i.e., pleated or layered, as the dressing will tighten when it dries.	Steripaste Zipzoc Viscopaste

- Use sterile equipment, fluids and dressing materials. Discard any with broken packaging or any that have passed their expiry date.
- Do not do wound dressings if you have any hand infections, boils, sore throat or runny nose.

  Never attempt complex dressings when you have not had appropriate training and been assessed as competent. If you are in any doubt refer back to the nurse.

1. Confirm the patient's identity and obtain informed consent before proceeding.
2. Check the care plan and patient notes from the previous appointment.
3. Prepare the patient so that they are comfortable and the area to be dressed is adequately exposed. If this involves taking off clothing, make sure the treatment area is private and the patient is provided with a dignity cover where necessary.
4. Put on gloves to remove the dressing. Alternatively you may ask the patient to remove the dressing themselves and offer the facility to decontaminate their hands afterwards. Another way to remove a dressing is by inserting your hand inside the bag provided in some dressing packs, to remove the dressing and then inverting the bag so that the dressing is contained inside. This can then be attached to the side of the trolley nearest to the patient and used as the bag to collect the dirty swabs, gloves, etc.
5. Remove gloves. Decontaminate hands.
6. Note the condition of the wound. Seek advice from the registered nurse if the wound shows signs of any problems or if the patient reports any concerns.
7. Prepare the clean trolley. Select the appropriate dressing pack if required. Peel open and gently drop the inside pack onto the upper surface of the trolley. Open the inside pack by touching the corners only so that your hands never come into direct contact with the inside of the pack.
8. Once the sterile field is opened out onto the upper level of the trolley, other sterile items such as the dressing, can be opened and gently dropped onto the field. Non sterile items such as irrigation pods, adhesive tape, etc., can be placed on the lower level of the trolley so that they are within reach when needed. If using saline in plastic pouches you will need a sterile gallipot for the fluid, a syringe to irrigate the wound and a swab to clean the pouch.
9. Decontaminate hands. Put on gloves.
10. Clean the wound if necessary by gently irrigating with warm tap water (Fernandez 2004) or sterile saline. Do not routinely clean wounds – they should only be cleaned if they are contaminated with foreign particles, slough or necrotic tissue. Never use gauze or cotton wool on wounds as these may leave fibres in the wound and delay the healing process. Only ever use these to clean around the wound.
11. Apply the dressing(s) according to the manufacturer's instructions, without touching the side that will be in contact with the wound.
12. Apply adhesive tape if necessary (check for allergies).
13. Dispose of dressing packs and contaminated equipment in the clinical waste bin, in line with your local policy.
14. Remove gloves and decontaminate your hands.
15. Make sure the patient has a new appointment if they are to be seen again and always advise them to return sooner if they are having any problems.
16. Document your actions and observations on the patient notes.

REMOVING SUTURES: THE PROCESS: PROTOCOL!

You can download the National Occupational Standard SFHCHS14, *Remove wound closure materials from individuals* to use as a checklist for your competencies (Skills for Health 2011).

You can purchase suture removal packs which include a sterile field, suture cutter, forceps, gauze and bag for used dressings, swabs, etc. Sharps should be disposed of in the sharps bin in accordance with local policy.

Steps 1–9 as above. Then proceed as follows:

1. The nurse should assess the wound prior to suture removal.
2. Remove alternate sutures to begin with in case the wound has not healed well, so that if it starts to open, there are still some sutures left in situ.
3. Remove the suture by pulling the knot up with forceps and then cutting underneath the knot closest to the skin and pulling the suture through.
4. If there are any problems during the procedure or the patient has any discomfort, always check with the registered nurse before proceeding.
5. Dispose of the sutures in the clinical waste bag and the stitch cutter in the sharps bin.
6. Apply a dry dressing if required.
7. Remove gloves and decontaminate hands.
8. Advise the patient to come back if they have any problems.
9. Document your actions and observations on the patient notes.

Now have a go at the quiz below. You can check back in the chapter if you have forgotten anything.

WOUND CARE QUIZ

1) What is the function of the epidermis?
2) What does haemostasis mean?
3) What do the platelets do?
4) How long does the inflammatory phase in wound healing last?
5) What happens during the proliferation/granulation phase?
6) If a wound heals by primary intention, what does this mean?
7) List five signs of infection.
8) Which parts of the wound should be sampled when performing a wound swab?
9) What type of wound would a hydrocolloid be suitable for?
10) What would you do if the patient was complaining of increased pain or exudate?

Using a framework for reflection (see Chapter 2), try reflecting on a consultation where you performed a wound dressing. How did it go and what did you learn?

Box 16.1. Factors that may delay healing

> Infection
>
> Presence of foreign object
>
> Inappropriate dressing / wrong size
>
> Poor dressing technique
>
> Poor nutrition
>
> Smoking
>
> Chronic disease such as diabetes, COPD, anaemia, depression, heart disease
>
> Poor circulation
>
> Poor mobility
>
> Social factors and environment
>
> Radiotherapy/chemotherapy
>
> Immunosuppression
>
> Pressure
>
> Medication
>
> Age

Box 16.2. Characteristics of the ideal wound dressing

- Comfortable and acceptable for the patient
- Keep pain to a minimum
- Maintain a moist environment where there is an open wound bed, when the wound is healing by secondary intention
- Remove excess exudate
- Allow the exchange of gases such as oxygen in from the air to promote healing and carbon dioxide out (waste product)
- Maintain the correct temperature to facilitate healing (not too hot or cold)
- Provide protection from further trauma
- Prevent the entry of microorganisms
- Leave no particles in the wound when it is removed
- Be easily removed without causing trauma / hindering the epithelialisation of the wound
- Be nonallergenic and nontoxic

17

Chaperoning

In recent years, the role of the chaperone in health care has been recognised as increasingly important for patients and health care providers alike. It is often performed badly leaving the health professional and patient open to abuse and so it is vital that all those who are to perform the role, understand the reason for it and are able to do it properly. This chapter will outline the history behind the current situation and will provide guidelines for healthcare workers who may be asked to perform this role in the future.

All healthcare professionals have become acutely aware of the need to protect themselves from allegations of malpractice in today's litigious society. Furthermore it has become clear that the title of 'doctor' or 'nurse' does not always guarantee protection for the patient. Consider the case of Harold Shipman (Smith 2005) who was a GP who murdered many elderly patients. Consider also the recent case of Jimmy Savile who so blatantly abused his position of trust as a hospital porter and used his status as a respected fundraising celebrity, to abuse children and vulnerable patients for many decades. It is an unfortunate fact of life that in any sector of society there will be people who will choose to abuse their positions of trust and respect in order to satisfy their own perverse needs. Gould (2006) writing about Shipman, argues that systems to protect the public and regulate the professions have been inadequate.

THE AYLING INQUIRY

In 2004 the Department of Health set up an independent investigation into how the NHS handled allegations about the conduct of a GP Clifford Ayling (DH 2004). He was convicted of thirteen counts of indecent assault on patients between 1991 and 1998. The report describes a "long history of continuing unease" regarding the GP's behaviour which was over familiar and unprofessional when performing intimate examinations. His colleagues appear to have ignored the warning signs and "reworked the truth" to make it more acceptable and had ultimately failed their patients. This investigation culminated in the Ayling Inquiry of 2004 and it is this that has been the catalyst for the increased awareness of the importance of the role of the chaperone. The report recommended that all patients should be offered a chaperone for intimate examinations and that each NHS Trust should create a chaperone policy, make it explicit to patients, and resource it accordingly. Despite this, research printed in the Postgraduate Medical Journal (Metcalf et al. 2010) suggested that most trusts have ignored the recommendations. They concluded that, "The current financial difficulties seen in many trusts may be placing a relative unimportance on the chaperone role." They also worry that the lack of chaperone policies "may have severe medico-legal repercussions in the future."

Most staff performing the role of chaperone today are still unlikely to have received any training in the role and are unlikely to appreciate the full importance of it.

WHAT IS A CHAPERONE?

There is no established single definition of the term chaperone. It originates from the fifteenth century when it meant "hood for a hawk" and later came to mean "a woman who protects a young single woman." In French, the word *chaperonner* means to cover with a hood and today the word is used in the sense of "protector" (Wai et al. 2008).

The Department of Health (DH 2004) define the word chaperone as:

'a third party of the same sex as the patient who has nothing to gain from misinterpretation of the facts'.

This definition is now a few years old but it is still appropriate to use today although care is needed in the interpretation of this if the patient is gay as they may then prefer a third party of the opposite sex. The NHS Clinical Governance Support Team Guidance (2005) describes the chaperone as *a safeguard for all parties and a witness to continuing consent of the procedure* but also stresses that they cannot be a guarantee of protection for either the examiner or examinee.

The chaperone can act as an advocate for the patient assessing their understanding and offering an explanation when necessary (RCN 2002). However, no matter how good the chaperone is this does not negate the need for good communication and an adequate explanation of the procedure by the health professional performing the examination.

When is a chaperone needed?

The most common reasons for needing a chaperone are:

- To offer the patient protection against verbal, physical, or sexual abuse and identify inappropriate behaviour
- To provide protection for the health worker against allegations of malpractice
- To support the patient by providing reassurance and physical and emotional comfort during an embarrassing "sensitive" examination
- To maintain the patient's dignity and self-respect
- Whenever the patient requests a chaperone
- Whenever the doctor feels a chaperone is necessary

A "sensitive" examination may denote one that involves examining the breasts, rectum, or genitalia but it could be used to describe any part of the body depending on the religion and cultural customs of the patient. Some authors argue that examination of the torso should also routinely be considered under the heading of intimate examination as cases of inappropriate behaviour during such examinations have generated huge concern (Wai et al. 2008). They question whether the current GMC guidelines offer enough protection for patients in all situations.

What if a patient declines to have a chaperone?

- It is important to document that the offer was made and declined.
- The healthcare professional may decline to examine the patient in this case if in their clinical judgement this would put them at risk of unjust or invalid accusation.

Sometimes a nurse or HCA will be asked to assist in a minor operation or procedure such as inserting a contraceptive coil. While assisting, they are expected to pass instruments to the doctor, write up forms and so on. The Medical Protection Society Guidelines (2012) consider this as a potential part of the role of chaperone. Whether or not they can fully support the patient when they are also assisting the doctor is however debatable, and I hope by the end of the chapter, you will agree with me that in terms of best practice, it is better to separate the role of chaperone from that of assistant.

Using a framework for reflection (see Chapter 2), try reflecting on a consultation where you were acting as a chaperone or alternatively where you have been chaperoned as a patient yourself. How did it go and what did you learn?

The HCA as chaperone

Before the Ayling Inquiry (DH 2004) there were very few, if any, recommendations as to who should act as a chaperone, and it would usually have been the nurse or female receptionist who was expected to perform the role. Friends or relatives may also have been considered as appropriate and indeed are still in the current General Medical Guidelines (GMC) guidelines (2006), but care is needed here to consider whether they may have anything to gain by misinterpreting the facts. For patients with learning difficulties a family member or carer may be the best person to act as chaperone, and in this instance a careful and sensitive explanation of the procedure is vital.

As a HCA, the role of chaperone may be one you can perform very competently providing you have the appropriate knowledge and understanding but you should have access to a nurse mentor to discuss any concerns. Furthermore you should ensure that there is a Chaperone Policy or Protocol in place so that all members of the team understand what the role entails. You may also be the best person to prepare an information poster for the waiting areas. The poster should outline the role and availability of chaperones and how patients can request one. Clear notices will reassure patients and increase understanding regarding the need of either doctor or patient to expect an extra degree of protection.

Chaperoning: The process

1. Introduce yourself to the patient.
2. Check that they have consented to your presence.
3. Give the patient privacy to undress and provide a dignity sheet to preserve their dignity.
4. Do not assist the patient with removal of their clothes unless they indicate that they need assistance.
5. Assist the patient onto the examining couch only when necessary and without putting yourself at risk of injury.
6. Only expose the area of the body required for the doctor to carry out the examination.
7. Maintain a position where you can observe the procedure at all times. This means you should always stand *inside* the curtains and usually at the head of the couch.
8. Check that the doctor has explained the procedure and that the patient understands what the examination will involve.
9. Keep the discussion relevant to the procedure and avoid unnecessary personal comments. Although it is sometimes tempting to discuss the weather or other topics in an attempt to relax the patient, this can have the effect of distracting the patient and chaperone and may make it more difficult for the patient to voice any concerns or discomfort.
10. Ensure the patient's dignity and privacy is respected as far as possible throughout the procedure.
11. Check for continuing consent if the patient appears to be uncomfortable or unhappy.
12. At the end of the examination allow the patient privacy to redress fully and only leave the room when they are fully dressed and before the doctor continues with the consultation.
13. Remember to observe infection control guidelines at all times.
14. Observe strict confidentiality and do not discuss the consultation or examination with any other members of staff except on a 'need to know' basis. If you have any concerns about the procedure, always discuss these with your nurse mentor and document them clearly.
15. The health care professional should document details of the examination including the presence (or absence) of a chaperone and their name and the information given. They should also document any reservations or concerns the patient or they themselves may have had.

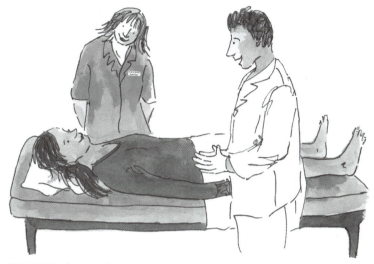

Figure 17.1 HCA chaperoning.

Consider this scenario

The doctor has asked you to act as chaperone for him to perform a breast examination (Figure 17.1). When you go into the room you realise that the patient is someone you know quite well, and she appears quite nervous and flustered when she sees you.

Dr. Jones quickly introduces you to the patient (Mrs. X) and asks you to stand just inside the curtain at the foot of the bed. Mrs. X takes off her blouse as instructed by the doctor but has some difficulty with the buttons so you help her. You make some small talk to try and relax her as she seems very tense – you ask about her children and chat about the recent bad weather. You also admire her all-over tan, all the time trying to relax Mrs. X.

Dr. Jones comes behind the curtain and stands between you and the patient. He asks Mrs. X to remove her bra and then proceeds to study her two breasts intently. He then asks Mrs. X to raise her hands above her head and then to put her hands on her hips all the while staring at her breasts. You're feeling a little embarassed by now so you look the other way and hope Mrs. X will notice that you're not staring as well.

Dr. Jones then proceeds to feel both Mrs. X's breasts as well as in the armpits and around the neck. Mrs. X is looking very red and uncomfortable and you do find yourself wondering why he needs to be so thorough when she only complained of a lump in one breast. Still he's the doctor and must know what he's doing.

While examining Mrs. X, Dr. Jones talks to you, commenting on how busy the surgery is and asking if you will get the notes out for the next patient when you go out.

The breast examination given in the scenario is exactly as it should be done but if this is not explained to the patient, it might seem a little odd.

When Dr. Jones has finished examining Mrs. X and before she puts her top back on, he thanks you for your help and suggests that you can now leave. You're glad to get out because you just find the whole thing so awkward.

- How do you think the patient would have felt in this scenario and why?
- Using the information given in the chapter, suggest some ways this experience could have been improved for the patient and safer in terms of protecting the doctor from allegations of malpractice.

Section V
Finishing Touches

18

Training for the Future

At the beginning of this book I talked a little about the evolving role of the HCA and what the future might hold in terms of regulation. Part of this process must be about compulsory training to a recognized standard so that everyone will understand what the term healthcare assistant means and what that person has achieved in terms of training and competence.

SO WHAT TYPE OF TRAINING SHOULD YOU LOOK FOR?

The training should incorporate mandatory topics including basic life support, health and safety, moving and handling, and should also include those skills and knowledge necessary to provide care for patients in a dignified and compassionate manner. Training should be competence-based, quality-assured, and assessed against nationally recognized standards such as the **National Occupational Standards** (RCN 2012a, Skills for Health 2011). It should also be set at an appropriate level to your needs within your place of work. You should have written evidence of your competence and this should be assessed at least annually and whenever the national guidelines on a particular task are changed as happened recently with blood pressure measurement. Most of the literature on training for HCAs now recommends that training should be in line with the NHS Knowledge and Skills Framework (NHS KSF 2004). This is a competence framework designed to support personal development and career progression within the NHS. It provides NHS KSF post outlines to identify the knowledge and skills that an individual needs to apply to their job and should help to identify any gaps in the knowledge and skills of the individual. It should also identify the learning and development that is needed to close that gap, usually through the deployment of a personal development plan that is developed in conjunction with the manager or appraiser.

At the moment, there is no standardization for training of HCAs, and most training occurs after you have been accepted for the role. Your employer should endeavour to make sure you are competent in the skills you need for your role and you should have an induction programme that includes training in all the basic skills. First Steps for HCAs is a useful online resource provided by the RCN (2013a) that outlines the role and gives an introduction to some of the core skills required.

Courses in health and social care starting at level 2 and progressing to level 3 and beyond are available in many local further education facilities and may provide relevant training depending on your proposed area of work. Some Trusts are also running Apprenticeships in Health where it is possible to earn whilst you learn. Information about these apprenticeships is available at some of the websites listed at the end of this chapter.

The Open University has a foundation degree programme in Healthcare Practice for HCAs who are already working, and it is open to HCAs without any formal qualifications. You can progress through this framework from the Certificate of Higher Education in Healthcare Practice to a full foundation degree. Other private organisations offer various healthcare assistant courses.

Always make sure that the training you sign up to is rigorous and accredited at the appropriate level for you (level 2, 3 or 4) depending on your role and experience.

If you are an experienced HCA working at a senior level or an assistant practitioner and you want to progress on to do your preregistration nurse education, you may be able to seek secondment from your current employer onto an appropriate programme at a local university, as a stepping stone to full registration.

Remember your initial training is just the start of your journey on a programme of lifelong learning. You should always strive to keep updated and make sure your competence remains valid and current in line with current evidence based guidelines. Your needs and the needs of the health- and social-care sector will be forever changing, and you can never stand still. The future for HCAs is a very interesting and exciting one, and there will always be more to learn as the role develops. Never take on any task where you have not had the necessary training and are not competent.

Keep learning and consolidating your knowledge and you can enjoy your role, happy in the knowledge that you are doing the best for your patients.

INSURANCE

Wherever you work, always make sure you are properly insured before you take on any clinical tasks. You may be insured under a group scheme in your place of work or you may need to seek separate cover. Specific organisations that offer insurance for healthcare assistants include the RCN, Unison, the Medical Protection Society and The Medical Defence Union.

Useful websites for training and insurance:

Access 2 Education (offers accredited training at Level 2 and 3 through Agored Cymru), http://www.access2education.co.uk/

Bradford Primary Care Training Centre (offers training accredited through Teeside University), http://www.primarycaretraining.co.uk/

Career and opportunities in NHS Scotland, https://jobs.scot.nhs.uk

HealthTrain (offers training accredited at Level 2 and 3 through Agored Cymru), http://www.healthtrain.co.uk

Health and social care in Northern Ireland, http://www.n-i.nhs.uk/

Health in Wales, http://www.wales.nhs.uk/

MDU, http://www.themdu.com/

MPS, http://www.medicalprotection.org/uk/

NHS, Careers http://www.nhscareers.nhs.uk/

Open University, http://www.open.ac.uk/

RCN, http://www.rcn.org.uk/

Unison, http://www.unison.org.uk/

Glossary

Adrenal insufficiency – a condition where the adrenal glands are unable to produce enough steroid hormones such as cortisol. This can be fatal if left untreated.

Alveolus – a tiny air filled sac at the end of the airways in the lungs. The alveoli are designed to maximise surface area for the exchange of oxygen and carbon dioxide.

Ambulatory blood pressure monitoring – a non invasive method of recording blood pressure over 24 hours while the patient goes about their normal activities. It is thought to provide an accurate reflection of blood pressure.

Anticoagulant – medication that reduces the ability of the blood to clot.

Anaemia – a condition where there are fewer red blood cells or less haemoglobin in each red blood cell. Haemoglobin attaches to oxygen so if there is less of it, the blood is not able to carry as much oxygen around the body.

Anaerobic – living without oxygen.

Aneurysm – a bulge in an artery wall where the wall is weakened and liable to rupture.

Angina – pain that comes from the heart. It occurs when the coronary arteries supplying the heart with blood become narrowed.

Anorexia – lack of appetite. Anorexia nervosa – an eating disorder characterised by distorted body image and an irrational fear of gaining weight.

Anterior – towards the front.

Antimicrobial – an agent that inhibits the growth of microorganisms or kills them.

Antimuscarinic – the term given to a group of drugs that are smooth muscle relaxants. They will help to dilate or open up the constricted airways in COPD.

Arrythmia – a problem with the rate or rhythm of the heart beat.

Arteriole – a very tiny artery, usually the terminal branch of the artery that connects to the capillary.

Atherosclerosis – a condition where the arteries are narrowed by fatty deposits called plaques or atheromas. The restricted blood flow can damage the affected organ (e.g. the heart) and stop it working properly.

Atrial fibrillation – an abnormal heart rhythm and a major cause of stroke.

Auscultatory – a method of listening to the sounds of the body such as from the heart or lungs, usually using a stethoscope.

Autopsy – examination of a dead body (cadaver) to determine the cause of death.

Axilla – the area under the arm. Also known as the armpit.

Bevel – the sloping point at the sharp end of the needle.

Bilirubin – the yellow pigment in bile produced when the liver breaks down old red blood cells.

Bronchodilator – a substance that dilates (opens up) the airways (bronchi and bronchioles) in the lungs.

Bronchus – the large air tube that begins at the end of the trachea and branches into the lungs.

Bundle of His – a bundle of modified heart muscle that transmits the electrical impulse from the atrio–ventricular node to the right and left ventricles.

Capillary – the smallest blood vessel where the wall is only one cell thick.

Catalyst – a substance that speeds up a chemical reaction.

Cellulitis – an infection of the deeper layers of the skin usually caused by Group A Streptococcus bacteria.

Contraindication – a condition or reason to withhold certain treatment.

Connective tissue – groups of tissue in the body that maintain the form of the body by supporting, anchoring and connecting the various parts of the body.

Cross contamination – the transfer of a contaminant from one source to another that may result in infection.

Cyanosis – a bluish discoloration of the skin and mucous membranes usually due to a lack of oxygen in the blood.

Debridement – the removal of dead damaged or infected tissue to enable the healing process.

Deep vein thrombosis (DVT) – the formation of a clot in a deep vein, usually in the leg. If a piece of the clot breaks off and travels to the lung, it can cause a pulmonary embolism which can be fatal.

Dehydration – a reduction in the normal water content of the body causing an upset in the delicate balance of minerals.

Diaphragm – a sheet of muscle that extends across the bottom of the rib cage separating the thorax from the abdomen.

Domiciliary – provided at home.

Doppler – ultrasound used to examine the blood flow in the major arteries and veins.

Efficacy – the capacity to produce a desired result or effect.

Electrolyte – substances found in the body that carry an electrical charge. They have to be present in the right amounts to maintain homeostasis for the proper functioning of the body.

Emphysema – a long-term lung disease where there is damage to the air sacs (alveoli) in the lungs.

Endocarditis – inflammation of the inner layer of the heart.

Enzyme – proteins that control the rate of chemical reactions in the body.

Epithelialisation – migration of newly formed skin cells across a wound bed during the healing process.

Erythrocyte – another name for a red blood cell.

Exacerbation – a worsening or flare up of symptoms.

Excoriation – tearing or wearing of skin cells usually due to rubbing or scratching.

Exfoliation – removal of the dead skin cells on the outermost surface of the skin.

Exudates – fluid such as pus or clear fluid leaking out of nearby blood vessels into surrounding tissues or wounds where there is inflammation or infection.

Fistula – an abnormal passage or connection between two organs or areas that do not normally connect. This can result from injury, surgery, infection or inflammation.

Fungating – a type of skin lesion characterised by ulceration and necrosis (death of tissue) usually caused by a cancerous growth breaking through the skin. There is usually a characteristic offensive odour.

Gallipot – a small plastic pot used for holding cleaning fluid, e.g., sodium chloride or water, that may be used during a wound dressing or a minor operation.

Genito – urinary tract – the system of organs concerned with the production and excretion of urine and those concerned with reproduction.

Haematological test – a blood test that provides information about the type, number and appearance of red and white blood cells and platelets.

Haematuria – blood in the urine.

Haemoglobin – a substance in red blood cells that combines with and carries oxygen around the body and gives the blood its red colour.

Haemophilia – a hereditary condition where the body is unable to control or stop bleeding when a blood vessel is injured.

Heart failure – a condition where the heart is unable to pump enough blood to meet the needs of the body.

Hydrophilic – water loving.

Hypercoaguability – a tendency of the blood to coagulate more quickly than normal increasing the risk of blood clots.

Hypergranulating – where tissue is progressing beyond the surface of the wound in the healing process.

Hyperlipidaemia – a high level of fat (cholesterol, low density lipoprotein and triglycerides) in the blood. An important risk factor for heart disease.

Hyper-responsiveness (of the airways) – a condition where the airways in the lungs get smaller (constrict) when exposed to a trigger or allergen.

Hyperthyroidism – a hormonal condition where the thyroid gland produces too much thyroxine which speeds up the body's metabolism.

Hypoallergenic – provokes fewer allergic reactions.

Hypoxia – a deficiency in the amount of oxygen that reaches the tissues of the body.

Immunosuppression – suppression of the body's immune system resulting in an inability to fight infection or disease.

Impermeable – not allowing fluid to pass through.

Inferior vena cava – the large vein that carries de-oxygenated blood from the lower half of the body back to the right side of the heart.

In situ – in position.

Insulin resistance – a condition where the cells fail to respond to the normal effects of insulin. May progress to Type 2 diabetes.

Intercostal space – the space between two ribs.

Intravenous – within a vein. Usually refers to giving medication or fluid through a tube or needle inserted into the vein.

Ischaemia – reduced blood supply depriving an area of essential oxygen and nutrients.

Ketoacidosis – a complication of diabetes where the body is unable to break down glucose because there is not enough insulin. It breaks down fat instead as a source of fuel and this causes the build-up of a by-product called ketones which can disrupt the body's metabolism.

Leukaemia – cancer of the blood or bone marrow.

Lipoprotein – molecules made of protein and fat that carry cholesterol and similar substances through the blood.

Low adherence – will not stick easily.

Lymph node clearance – removal of lymph nodes from the arm pit to check if cancer has spread into the nodes and help determine if further treatment is needed and also to eliminate any cancerous nodes.

Maceration – a process where the skin is softened and broken down by extended exposure to wetness or moisture.

Malaise – a generalised feeling of discomfort or illness, feeling unwell.

Malpractice – negligence or incompetence on the part of a professional.

Metabolic rate – the rate at which the body burns calories.

Mid clavicular line – an imaginary vertical line crossing through the right or left clavicle (collar bone) to the hip bone.

Mitral valve – a valve made up of a dual flap of skin situated between the left atrium and left ventricle in the heart. It allows blood to flow into the right ventricle when the right atrium contracts but prevents the back flow of blood when the ventricle contracts.

Mucolytic – a medicine that makes sputum less thick and sticky and easier to cough up.

Myocardial infarction – a heart attack resulting from an interruption in the blood supply to an area of heart muscle causing the heart cells to be damaged or die.

Necrotic – death of cells or tissues through injury or disease where there is an inadequate blood supply. It is irreversible.

Opiate analgesic – a class of drugs derived from the opium poppy that are used to relieve moderate to severe pain.

Orthostatic – related to or caused by standing up.

Palpable – able to be touched or felt.

Palliative – an area of healthcare focused on relieving pain and suffering, to promote quality of life and manage end of life symptoms.

Pathogen – a microorganism capable of causing disease in its host.

Pericardial tamponade – a collection of fluid in the pericardial sac around the heart. It interferes with the performance of the heart and will cause death if left untreated.

Peripheral vascular disease – a condition where a build-up of fatty deposits in the arteries restricts the blood supply to the leg muscles.

Pneumothorax – a collection of air in the pleural space around the lungs resulting in collapse of the lung on the affected side.

Polycythaemia – a condition where there are too many red blood cells in the blood resulting in increased thickness or stickiness of the blood reducing blood flow to the organs of the body and sometimes resulting in clots.

Posterior – further back in position.

Postural hypotension – a reduction of at least 20mm Hg systolic and at least 10mm Hg diastolic blood pressure within three minutes of standing upright. A common cause of falls in the elderly.

Pre-eclampsia – a medical condition characterised by high blood pressure and protein in the urine that occurs during pregnancy with risk of serious complications to mother and baby.

Proteinurea – the abnormal presence of protein in the urine in detectable quantities usually defined as an excess of 300mg protein per day. There are many possible causes but persistent proteinurea should be investigated.

Pulmonary embolism – a blockage in a blood vessel in the lungs which can cause collapse and death.

Pyelonephritis – a kidney infection.

Renal artery stenosis – narrowing of the renal artery (the artery that supplies the kidney with blood) that may lead to impaired kidney function.

Sick sinus syndrome – a collection of conditions where there is malfunction of the sinus node resulting in arrhythmia.

Slough – a layer of dead tissue separated from surrounding living tissue that can result in delayed healing. It is made up of dead cells that have accumulated in the exudate and is typically a white/yellow colour.

Statins – a class of drugs used to lower cholesterol.

Sternal border – the long edge of the breast bone.

Superior vena cava – the large vein that carries de-oxygenated blood from the upper half of the body back to the right side of the heart.

Supine – lying down with the face up.

Systemic – affecting the entire body.

Thyrotoxicosis – a disease caused by excessive concentrations of thyroid hormones in the body.

Trachea – the large airway that leads from the larynx (voice box) to the bronchi (large airways at the top of the lungs). Also known as the wind pipe.

Tricuspid valve – a three segmented valve that stops blood in the right ventricle from flowing back into the right atrium.

Turbid – having sediment or particles stirred up or suspended in fluid, clouded, opaque.

Varicose eczema – a type of eczema caused by increased pressure in the veins that affects the legs. Pigment from the blood leaks into the skin causing discoloration, inflammation and ulceration.

Venuole – a very small blood vessel that allows blood to return from the capillaries to the veins.

References

1. Access to Health Records Act 1990. http://www.legislation.gov.uk/ukpga/1990/23 (accessed January 12, 2013).

2. Allegranzi, B., Pittet, D. 2009. Role of hand hygiene in healthcare-associated infection prevention. *Journal of Hospital Infection* 73(4) 305–15

3. ASH 2012. The economics of tobacco. http://ash.org.uk/files/documents/ASH_121.pdf (accessed December 10, 2012).

4. Beach, M.C., Keruly J., Moore R.D. 2006. Is the quality of the patient provider relationship associated with better adherence and health outcomes for patients with HIV? *J Gen Intern Med* 21:661–665

5. Beech, M. 2007. Confidentiality in health care: conflicting legal and ethical issues. *Nursing Standard Vol* 21, No. 21, 42–46.

6. Bolton, G. 2010. *Reflective Practice. Writing and professional development* (3rd ed). SAGE publications.

7. Borg, J. 2010. *Body Language: 7 Easy Lessons to Master the Silent Language.* FT Press

8. BBC News 2013. Consider tougher regulation in obesity fight – Labour http://www.bbc.co.uk/news/health-20914685

9. British Cardiovascular Society 2010 Clinical Guidelines by Consensus. Recording a Standard 12 Lead Electrocardiogram. An Approved Methodology. http://www.scst.org.uk/resources/consensus_guideline_for_recording_a_12_lead_ecg_Rev_072010b.pdf (accessed June 6, 2012).

10. British Heart Foundation 2011. *Apple or pear, do we need to care?* http://www.bhf.org.uk/media/news-from-the-bhf/obesity-and-body-shape.aspx (accessed November 10, 2013)

11. British Heart Foundation 2012. Physical Activity Supplement http://www.bhf.org.uk/publications/view-publication.aspx?ps=1001983 (accessed November 10, 2013).

12. British Hypertension Society 2012. *Blood Pressure Monitors validated for home/clinical use* http://www.bhsoc.org//index.php?cID=247 (accessed June 12, 2012).

13. BTS SIGN 2012. *British Guideline on the Management of Asthma 101* http://www.brit-thoracic.org.uk/Portals/0/Guidelines/AsthmaGuidelines/sign101%20Jan%202012.pdf (accessed August 20, 2012).

14. Bulman, C., Schutz, S. 2004 (Eds) *Reflective Practice in Nursing* Blackwell Scientific Publications

15. Chapman, A., Law, S. 2009. Bridging the gap: an innovative dementia learning program for health care assistants in hospital wards using facilitator-led discussions *International Psychogeriatrics* 21:Supplement 1 S58–S63

16. Clever, S., Jin, L., Levinson, W., Meltzer, D. 2008. Does Doctor–Patient Communication Affect Patient Satisfaction with Hospital Care? Results of

an Analysis with a Novel Instrumental Variable http://www.ncbi.nlm.nih.gov/pmc/articles/PMC2653895/ (accessed September 2, 2013).

17. Clinical Knowledge Summaries 2012. Hypercalcaemia management. http://www.cks.nhs.uk/hypercalcaemia/management/scenario_diagnosis_and_assessment/view_full_scenario (accessed August 12, 2012).

18. Collier, M. 2004. Recognition and management of wound infections http://www.worldwidewounds.com/2004/january/Collier/management-of-Wound-Infections.html (accessed September 3, 2012).

19. Computer Misuse Act 1990. http://www.legislation.gov.uk/ukpga/1990/18/contents (accessed January 12, 2013).

20. Cooper, R. 2010. Ten top tips for taking a wound swab *Wounds International* http://www.woundsinternational.com/practice-development/ten-top-tips-for-taking-a-wound-swab (accessed January 9, 2013).

21. Data Protection Act 1998. http://www.legislation.gov.uk/ukpga/1998/29/contents (accessed January 12, 2013).

22. Department of Health 2003. Confidentiality: NHS Code of Practice. The Stationery Office, London.

23. Department of Health 2008. The Health and Social Care Act. http://www.dh.gov.uk/en/Publicationsandstatistics/Legislation/Actsandbills/HealthandSocialCareBill/index.htm (accessed June 30, 2013).

24. Department of Health 1997. The Caldicott Report http://webarchive.nationalarchives.gov.uk/+/www.dh.gov.uk/en/Publicationsandstatistics/Publications/PublicationsPolicyAndGuidance/DH_4068403 (accessed January 12, 2013).

25. Department of Health 2004. Committee of inquiry: independent investigation into how the NHS handled allegations about the conduct of Clifford Ayling. http://www.dh.gov.uk/en/Publicationsandstatistics/Publications/PublicationsPolicyAndGuidance/DH_4088996 (accessed January 2, 2013).

26. Department of Health 2011a. Enabling Excellence: Autonomy and Accountability for Health and Social Care Staff http://www.dh.gov.uk/en/Publicationsandstatistics/Publications/PublicationsPolicyAndGuidance/DH_124359 (accessed November 12, 2012).

27. Department of Health 2011b. *An Outcomes Strategy for Chronic Obstructive Pulmonary Disease and Asthma in England* http://www.dh.gov.uk/prod_consum_dh/groups/dh_digitalassets/documents/digitalasset/dh_128428.pdf (accessed August 10, 2012).

28. Dougherty, L., Lister, S. 2007 *The Royal Marsden Manual of clinical Nursing Procedures.* Blackwell Publishing.

29. Driscoll, J. 2007. Practising Clinical Supervision: A Reflective Approach for Healthcare Professionals (2nd ed) Balliere Tindall Elsevier.

30. Elhassan, H.A., Dixon, T. 2011. MRSA contaminated venepuncture tourniquets in clinical practice *Postgrad Med Journal* doi:10.1136 http://pmj.bmj.com/content/early/2012/01/31/postgradmedj-2011-130411.abstract (accessed August 10, 2012).

31. Freedom of Information Act 2000. http://www.legislation.gov.uk/ ukpga/2000/36/contents (accessed January 12, 2013).

32. General Medical Council 2006 *Maintaining boundaries – guidance for doctors.* http://www.gmc-uk.org/guidance/ethical_guidance/maintaining_ boundaries.asp (accessed January 10, 2013).

33. Gibbs, G. 1988. Learning by Doing: A Guide to Teaching and Learning. London: Further Educational Unit.

34. Godlee, F. 2011. What is Health? *BMJ* 343:d4817.

35. Hand, T. 2011. Applying HCA Resources to general practice. *Practice Nursing* 22 (12) 658–660.

36. Hassan Arshad, S. et al. 2012. The effect of parental allergy on childhood allergic diseases depends on the sex of the child *The Journal of Allergy and Clinical Immunology* http://www.jacionline.org/article/S0091- 6749(12)00611-2/abstract (accessed October 12, 2012).

37. Health and Safety Executive 2010. *Healthcare.* http://www.hse.gov.uk/ biosafety/healthcare.htm (accessed June 30, 2013).

38. Health and Safety Executive 2013. Control of substances hazardous to health (COSHH). http://www.hse.gov.uk/coshh/index.htm (accessed January 31, 2013).

39. Health Professions Wales 2004. Health Care Support Workers. All Wales Scoping Project Final Report. http://www.wales.nhs.uk/sites3/ Documents/484/HCSW%20All%20Wales%20Scoping%20Project%20 -%20Final%20 Report%20Pages%201%20to%20155.pdf (accessed November 12, 2012).

40. Health Protection Agency 2012. *MRSA rates slashed but other bugs a threat.* http://www.nhs.uk/news/2012/05may/Pages/mrsa-hospital-acquired- infection-rates.aspx (accessed July 12, 2013).

41. Human, R.P., Jones, G.A. 2004. Evaluation of swab transport systems against a published standard. *Journal of Clinical Pathology* 57: 762–3.

42. Jasper, M. 2003. *Beginning Reflective Practice* Nelson Thornes Ltd.

43. Kelly, F. 2003. Infection control: validity and reliability in wound swabbing. *British Journal Nursing* 12 (16) 959–64.

44. Kessler I., Heron P., Dopson S., Magee H., Swain D., Ashkam. J, 2010. The Nature and consequences of support workers in a hospital setting: final report, London: NHS Institute for Health Research.

45. Kligfield Gettes, L.S., Bailey, J.J *2007. Recommendations for the Standardisation and interpretation of the electrocardiogram: part 1/ Circulation.* 115:10 1306–1324.

46. Lee, K., Bacon, L. 2010. Social networking: confidentiality and professional issues. *British Journal of Midwifery.* 18: 8 533–534.

47. Lindenfield, G. 2001. *Simple Steps to Getting What You Want.* Thorsens.

48. Local Authority Coordinators of Regulatory Services 2007. *LACORS Medical weighing project* http://www.westcoweigh.co.uk/PDFs/Medical- Weighing.pdf.

49. Ludwick. R., Silva, M. 2000. Ethics; Nursing Around the World: Cultural Values and Ethical Conflicts. *Online Journal of Issues in Nursing* 5(3)

50. Lustig, R. 2012. *Fat Chance* Fourth Estate.

51. McGilton, K., Irwin-Robinson, H., Boscart, V., Spanjevic, L. 2006. Communication enhancement: nurse and patient satisfaction outcomes in a complex continuing care facility. *Journal of Advanced Nursing* 54 (1): 35–44.

52. Medical protection Society 2012. *Chaperones* http://www.medicalprotection.org/uk/england-factsheets/chaperones (accessed January 12. 2013).

53. Mental Capacity 2005. Act http://www.legislation.gov.uk/ukpga/2005/9/contents (accessed January 12, 2013).

54. Mental Health Act 2007. http://www.legislation.gov.uk/ukpga/2007/12/contents (accessed January 12, 2013).

55. Metcalf, N., Moores, K., Murhy, N. Pring, D. 2010 The extent to which chaperone policies are used in acute hospital trusts in England. *Postgraduate Medical Journal* 86 636–40 http://pmj.bmj.com/content/86/1021//636.short (accessed January 15, 2013).

56. Michel, F. 2008. *Assert Yourself.* Perth, Western Australia: Centre for Clinical Interventions. http://www.cci.health.wa.gov.au/docs/Assertmodule%207.pdf (accessed November 10, 2013).

57. Mid Staffordshire NHS Foundation Trust 2013. The Francis Report http://www.midstaffspublicinquiry.com/report (accessed February 28, 2013).

58. NHS Choices 2011a. *The eatwell plate.* http://www.nhs.uk/Livewell/Goodfood/Pages/eatwell-plate.aspx (accessed January 2, 2013).

59. NHS Choices 2011b. *Physical activity guidelines for adults.* http://www.who.int/dietphysicalactivity/pa/en/index.html (accessed January 2, 2013).

60. NHS Choices 2012. *10 health benefits of stopping smoking.* http://www.nhs.uk/livewell/smoking/Pages/betterlives.aspx?WT.mc_id=31001 (accessed December 12, 2013).

61. NHS & Community Care Act 1990. http://www.legislation.gov.uk/ukpga/1990/19/contents (accessed January 5, 2013).

62. NHS Education for Scotland 2010. Health Care Support Workers. The Development of the Clinical Health Care Support Worker Role: A Review of the Evidence. NES, Edingburgh.

63. NHS Institute for Innovation and Improvement 2008. Protocol Based Care. http://www.institute.nhs.uk/quality_and_service_improvement_tools/quality_and_service_improvement_tools/protocol_based_care.html (accessed January 24, 2013).

64. NHS Knowledge and Skills Framework 2004. *The NHS KSF and the development review process.* http://www.dh.gov.uk/en/Publicationsandstatistics/Publications/PublicationsPolicyAndGuidance/DH_4090843 (accessed May 10, 2012).

65. NHS Professionals 2010. Record Keeping Guidelines Clinical Governance. http://www.nhsprofessionals.nhs.uk (accessed January 12, 2013).

66. National Heart Lung and Blood Institute 2003. *The Seventh Report of the Joint National Committee on Prevention, Detection, Evaluation and Treatment of High Blood Pressure JNC7.* http://www.nhlbi.nih.gov/guidelines/hypertension/jnc7full.pdf (accessed July 2, 2012).

67. National Institute for Health and Clinical Excellence 2004. The guideline development process, an overview for stakeholders, the public and the NHS. NICE, London.

68. National Institute for Health and Clinical Excellence 2006a. Brief interventions and referral for smoking cessation (PH1). http://www.nice.org.uk/PHI001 (accessed January 10, 2013).

69. National Institute for Health and Clinical Excellence 2006b. Obesity (CG43). http://guidance.nice.org.uk/CG43 (accessed December 12, 2013).

70. National Institute for Health and Clinical Excellence 2010. Chronic Heart Failure. (CG108) http://www.nice.org.uk/CG108 (accessed June 14, 2012).

71. National Institute for Health and Clinical Excellence 2011a *Hypertension (CG127)*. http://guidance.nice.org.uk/CG127 (accessed June 12, 2012).

72. National Institute for Health and Clinical Excellence 2011b. *Chronic Obstructive Pulmonary disease (COPD) (QS10)*. http://guidance.nice.org.uk/QS10 (accessed September 14, 2012).

73. National Institute for Health and Clinical Excellence 2012. Infection control (CG139). http://guidance.nice.org.uk/CG139 (accessed May 3, 2013).

74. National Society for the Prevention of Cruelty to Children NSPCC 2012. Gillick Competency and Fraser Guidelines Factsheet. http://www.nspcc.org.uk/inform/research/questions/gillick_wda61289.html (accessed January 2, 2013).

75. Nursing and Midwifery Council 2008. The Code: Standards of Conduct Performance and Ethics for Nurses and Midwives. NMC, London.

76. Nursing and Midwifery Council 2009. Record Keeping Guidance for Nurses and Midwives. http://www.nmc-uk.org/Documents/NMC-Publications/NMC-Record-Keeping-Guidance.pdf (accessed January 3, 2013).

77. Nursing and Midwifery Council 2012. Consent. www.nmc-uk.org/Nurses-and-midwives/Regulation-in-practice/Regulation-in-practice- Topics/consent/ (accessed January 3, 2013).

78. O'Donnell, M. (2009) Definition of Health Promotion. *American Journal of Health Promotion* 24:1. pp iv.

79. Oelofsen, N. 2012. *Developing Reflective Practice: A Guide for Students and Practitioners of Health and Social Care* Scion Publishing Ltd

80. Patient.co.uk 2010 *MRSA* www.patient.co.uk/health/MRSA.htm (accessed April 3, 2013).

81. Patient.co.uk 2012. *Healthy Eating.* http://www.patient.co.uk/health/Healthy-Eating.htm (accessed January 3, 2013).

82. Pendergast, J. 2002. Why you weigh more on thick carpet. http://www.inference.phy.cam.ac.uk/is/papers/bathroom_scales.pdf (accessed May 24, 2012).

83. Prochaska, J.O. and Di Clemente,C.C 1992. *Stages of Change and the modification of problem behaviours.* In Hersen, M., Eisler, R.M. and Miller, P.M. (Eds), Progress in behaviour modification. Sycamore: Sycamore Press.

84. Royal College of Nursing 2007. The Regulation of Healthcare Support Workers. Policy Briefing 11/2007. http://bit.ly/tkYddv (accessed 21 November 2012).

85. Royal College of Nursing 2009. *The Assistant Practitioner role: a Policy Discussion Paper. Policy briefing 06/2009.* http://bit.ly/vJklIc (accessed 21November 2012).

86. Royal College of Nursing 2011. Accountability and delegation: What you need to know. https://www.rcn.org.uk/__data/assets/pdf_file/0003/381720/003942.pdf (accessed February 10, 2013).

87. Royal College of Nursing 2012a. Position statement on the education and training of health care assistants. http://www.rcn.org.uk/__data/assets/pdf_file/0003/441912/Position_statement_-_HCAs_Final_V3.pdf (accessed February 10, 2013).

88. Royal College of Nursing 2012b. Record Keeping –the facts. Quick reference guide. http://www.rcn.org.uk/__data/assets/pdf_file/0005/476753/Record_keeping_cards_V5.pdf.

89. Royal College of Nursing 2012c. Wipe it Out. Essential Practice for Infection Prevention and Control. http://www.rcn.org.uk/_data/assets/pdf_file/0008/427832/004166.pdf.

90. Royal College of Nursing 2013a. First Steps for Health Care Assistants. http://rcn.org.uk/firststeps (accessed March 2, 2013).

91. Royal College of Nursing 2013b. First steps for Health Care Assistants. Verbal Communication. http://rcnhca.org.uk/communication/communication-methods/verbal-communication/ (accessed February 9, 2013).

92. Scottish Government 2010. *Healthcare support workers – mandatory standards and codes.* Scottish Government. http://www.scotland.gov.uk/Resource/Doc/288853/0088360.pdf (accessed January 10, 2013).

93. Skills for Health 2010. Key elements of the career framework. http://www.skillsforhealth.org.uk/about-us/resource-library/doc_details/301-career-framework-key-elements.html (accessed February 10, 2013).

94. Skills for Health 2011. Competencies / National Occupational Standards Available at http://www.skillsforhealth.org.uk/about-us/competences%10national-occupational-standards/

95. Skills for Health 2012. *Perform hand hygiene to prevent the spread of infection.* https://tools.skillsforhealth.org.uk/competence/show/html/id/3309/ (accessed December 20, 2012).

96. Smith M.J. 1975. *When I Say No, I Feel Guilty.* http://www.transcendedu.com/upload/when-i-say-no-i-feel-guilty-smith-e.pdf (accessed November 12, 2012).

97. Teare, L., Cookson, B., Stone, S. 2001. Hand Hygiene *BMJ* 323: 411–412.

98. Tingle, J. McHale, J. 2007. *Law and Nursing* Elsevier.

99. Wai, D., Katsaris, M., Singhal, R. 2008. Chaperones: are we protecting patients? *British Journal of General Practice* 58(546): 54–7. http://www.ncbi.nlm.nih.gov/pmc/articles/PMC2148245/ (accessed December 13, 2012).

100. Welch Allyn 2008. *Blood Pressure Training Manual. Evolution of BPM technology* p16. http://www.welchallyn.com/documents/Blood%20 Pressure%20Management/7171WAWorkbook_AUG5.pdf (accessed August 8, 2012).

101. Welsh Assembly Government WAG 2011. *Code of Conduct for healthcare support workers in Wales* Cardiff: Welsh Assembly Government. http://www.wales.nhs.uk/sitesplus/documents/829/ Final%20-%20NHS%20HSW%20Booklet%20ENG.pdf (accessed January 12, 2013).

102. Williams, B., Lindholm, L.H., Sever, P. 2008. Systolic Pressure is all that matters. *Lancet* 371:2219–2221.

103. World Health Organisation 1948. Preamble to the Constitution of the World Health Organization as adopted by the International Health Conference, New York, 19–22 June, 1946; signed on 22 July 1946 by the representatives of 61 States (Official Records of the World Health Organization, no. 2, p. 100) and entered into force on 7 April 1948.

104. World Health Organisation 2009. WHO guidelines for hand hygiene in health care. World Health Organization Press.

105. World Health Organisation 2010. WHO Guidelines on drawing blood: Best practices in phlebotomy. http://whqlibdoc.who.int/ publications/2010/9789241599221_eng.pdf (accessed August 4, 2012).

106. World Health Organisation 2013. WHO Global strategy on diet, physical activity and health. http://www.who.int/dietphysicalactivity/pa/en/index. html (accessed February 14, 2013).

Index